Susan Green

KETO DIET FOR BEGINNERS

6 DAYS TO ACT, THE LAST TO DARE. EXERCISE, FOOD, TIPS TO LOSE WEIGHT.

By

SUSAN GREEN

Contents

INTRODUCTION

Everybody's doing the keto diet. It's a cultural craze that's captured our imagination.

But let's remember that the ketogenic diet is a medical, or therapeutic, diet. So while it's extremely beneficial for people with certain conditions, it's not for everyone.

What do you eat on the keto diet?

The keto diet is essentially a high-fat diet — your meals are 70 or 80 percent fat; about 20 percent protein; and about 5 percent carbohydrate. It is not an Atkins high-protein diet.

Eating fat does not make your insulin go up, as eating carbs or protein does. So the keto diet does not spike your insulin, and you don't store fat. Instead, you burn it, creating the ketones that give you an effective and efficient metabolic jolt.

The keto diet switches you from burning glucose (which carbs provide) to burning ketones (which fat produces) for energy. When you do this, interesting things happen:

- Your metabolism speeds up.
- Your hunger goes away.
- Your muscle mass increases.
- Your blood pressure and heart disease risk profile improve.

What is Keto Diet?

The Keto diet emphasizes weight loss through fat-burning. The goal is to quickly lose weight and ultimately feel fuller with fewer cravings, while boosting your mood, mental focus and energy. According to Keto proponents, by slashing the carbs you consume and instead filling up on fats, you safely enter a state of ketosis. That's when the body breaks down both dietary and stored body fat into substances called ketones.

Your fat-burning system now relies mainly on fat – instead of sugar – for energy. While similar in some ways to familiar low-carb diets, the Keto diet's extreme carb restrictions – about 20 net carbs a day or less, depending on the version – and the deliberate shift into ketosis are what set this increasingly popular diet apart.

Benefits of a Ketogenic Diet

There are numerous benefits that come with being on keto: from weight loss and increased energy levels to therapeutic medical applications. Most anyone can safely benefit from eating a low-carb, high-fat diet. Below, you'll find a short list of the benefits you can receive from a ketogenic diet.

Insulin Resistance

Insulin resistance can lead to type II diabetes if left unmanaged. An abundant amount of research shows that a low carb, ketogenic diet can help people lower their insulin levels to healthy ranges.

Weight Loss

The ketogenic diet essentially uses your body fat as an energy source – so there are obvious weight loss benefits. On keto, your insulin (the fat storing hormone) levels drop greatly which turns your body into a fat burning machine.

Scientifically, the ketogenic diet has shown better results compared to low-fat and high-carb diets; even in the long term.

Many people incorporate MCT Oil into their diet (it increases ketone production and fat loss) by drinking ketoproof coffee in the morning.

Control Blood Sugar

Keto naturally lowers blood sugar levels due to the type of foods you eat. Studies even show that the ketogenic diet is a more effective way to manage and prevent diabetes compared to low-calorie diets.

If you're pre-diabetic or have Type II diabetes, you should seriously consider a ketogenic diet. We have many readers that have had success with their blood sugar control on keto.

Mental Focus

Many people use the ketogenic diet specifically for the increased mental performance.

Ketones are a great source of fuel for the brain. When you lower carb intake, you avoid big spikes in blood sugar. Together, this can result in improved focus and concentration.

Eggs on a Ketogenic Diet

There are many kinds of diets and nutrition that can be found either online, or in other sources. Many of them are based on a process called ketosis, in which your body stops using carbs as the primary source of energy, and instead uses fats as the main energy source. This state of ketosis can be achieved by a ketogenic diet, which is actually just another name for a low carbohydrate diet, because on the ketogenic diet, your goal is to eat food rich in proteins and fats, and low in carbohydrates. There are many things you can eat in order to meet the mentioned criteria.

Eggs have important and valuable nutritional properties. They are a great source of proteins. Chicken eggs, that are the most commonly eaten eggs have all the essential amino acids that are necessary humans, and also have many vitamins and minerals, like vitamin A, vitamin B6, vitamin B12, riboflavin, folic acid, and minerals like iron, calcium and potassium. Their high protein content is valued especially by many athletes and body builders that wish to increase their muscle mass, or maintain the current level.

On 100 grams of whole eggs, we have about 13 grams of proteins, 10 grams of fat and 1 gram of carbohydrates. An avarage chicken egg can have between 50 and 70 grams, so the amounts of proteins, fats or carbs can easily be calculated. Thereby if we take 60 grams as the weight of an avarage egg, it would contain around 8 grams of proteins, 6 grams of fat, and only around half a gram of carbs.

As we can see, the eggs have a very low amount of carbohydrates, and a high amount of fats and proteins, which is exactly what one needs to maintain the state of ketosis on a ketogenic diet. There are many recipes based on eggs which one can eat on a ketogenic diet, but one one should only make sure that nothing that contains carbs is added.

Are You Fooling or Fueling Your Body?

Year in and year out, people promise themselves that this is the year they will start exercising and losing weight. However, that journey is much more complex that many people think. Losing weight and taking care of your health also includes nutrition. If you go to the gym and do cardio, lift weights or even group exercise classes you will not see a change in your overall physique if you don't provide your body with the necessary fuel to make that change happen. The marriage between nutrition and exercise could make the difference in making this year the year that your life changes.

During Anaerobic exercise (resistance training) your body uses up muscle glycogen (a carbohydrate) in order to find energy sources of ATP (adenosine triphosphate). In high intensity exercises the body's glycogen can be depleted quite quickly due to the small amount found in the muscle. Due to this decline, blood sugars drop leaving you at risk of a poor workout and it can even influence your next one. Therefore, post workout, your body needs to replenish these glycogen stores in order to prepare your body for your next workout.

Think about what are you eating now? Do you know if you are supporting a change in your physique or hindering it by neglecting to add the right things into your diet? Are you incorporating healthy fats, carbohydrates and lean protein in your diet? Your body needs macronutrients to provide it with calories and energy for functioning. Macronutrients are classified as carbohydrates, fats, and protein. All of these macronutrients are essential and provide you with various amounts of energy in calories. Carbohydrates provide the body with 4 calories per gram, Protein 4 calories per gram, fats 9 calories per gram and ethanol-in alcoholic beverage form-delivers 7 calories per gram. Adding the right macronutrients into your body-along with a smart exercise/training program-can help you lose FAT weight and hold onto or even gain lean muscle. However, neglecting to add these macronutrients in the right amounts-or NOT engaging in an exercise training program-could lead to fat loss and muscle loss, which is a less than desirable result.

Many of you know the importance of eating macronutrient rich foods to support your exercise but what about supplemental forms of them? Food should always be your first resort however there are certain situations when supplements can benefit your workout and maximize your results more efficiently.

Protein shakes are a common supplement used at the gym post workout. One of the main reasons for having a protein shake at the end of your workout is to replenish the body and support the rebuilding of muscles that have been broken down during resistance/weight or endurance training. Another reason to have protein in the form of a shake after a workout is because it is a lot faster to make and consume than eating a meal (unless maybe you have a meal already prepared and can quickly swallow large chunks of food!). However, protein drinks should not be the only element of your post-workout drink.

When your body becomes efficient at creating and using energy for fuel, you begin to burn fat as well for energy. You do not exhaust all of your muscle fat during exercise and therefore you do not need to replace fat after a workout, especially if you are doing resistance training or short duration (less than several hours) endurance training or racing. However, it is important to maintain a diet with a modest amount of healthy fats.

Another great supplement that can be incorporated into your workout is a patented, sugar-free carbohydrate called Vitargo. Vitargo is a research based "supercarb"-an extract of starch-which has been studied in prestigious university laboratories. The subjects who took the Vitargo increased their work output by up to 23% just 2 hours after completing exhaustive exercise, compared to when they took a maltodextrin and sugars drink, or calorie-free placebo. Vitargo also doesn't cause the common bloating that occurs after ingesting other carbohydrates because it has been shown to move through the stomach and into the intestines 2.3x faster than a combo of maltodextrin and sugars (over 90% maltodextrin).That means you will get the necessary fuel you need for your muscles without experiencing that "heaviness", when taken pre-, during ("intra-"), or post-workout. Vitargo also has been researched to show that it replenishes glycogen stores 1.7 times faster than a maltodextrin plus sugars combo-again 2 hours after exhaustive exercise. Glycogen is the body's way of storing carbohydrates, like plants and grains store starch. It does this in muscles, and the liver and brain. This means you will be able to provide your body with the necessary fuel/energy replenishments needed for your next workout. In addition to all of these bonuses, Vitargo also increases the rate of blood sugar rise 2 times quicker compared to Maltodextrin and sugars.

So, what does all this mean? In order to get maximum results from your workout you need to be eating adequate amounts of macronutrients like carbohydrates, fats, and proteins every 3-4 hours in order to provide your body with the necessary energy and rebuilding components. You also, however, need to make sure that you are also giving your body the right supplements pre and post workout. Because of the unique nature of Vitargo, you can drink it pre-workout to provide your muscles and your brain with the necessary fuel you need to make it through an intense workout. You can also mix it with your protein powder post workout to replenish your glycogen stores, support muscle repair, and promote faster recovery before the next time you dive into an intense workout.

Providing your body with the necessary fuel pre and post workout, can not only bring yourself one step closer to your fitness goals but also fuel your workouts, not "fool" them! Next time I'll write about why many find it hard to train/work out while on a low carb or "keto" diet and how to use pulsed fueling tactics to have better workouts... and better results!

Painless Ways to Cut Carbs

The Atkins diet achieved peak fad status in 2004, and although it's since been replaced by trendy new ways of losing weight, it's had a lasting impact on how people view weight loss. Atkins recommended that dieters reduce their intake of carbohydrates. But that can be harder than it sounds. Here are some easy ways to cut carbs from your diet without sacrificing all of your favorite foodstuffs.

Substitute Your Spaghetti

A spiralizer is the kitchen invention you never knew you needed-and it's shockingly affordable, with many going for under $30. This nifty gadget can transform squash, zucchini, and other low-carb veggies into spaghetti (or other shapes), making a great substitute for that carb-heavy pasta you miss eating.

Skip the Starch

While you need veggies to stay healthy on your low-carb diet, you want to avoid the starchier varieties. Potatoes are an obvious no-go, but so are sweet potatoes, despite being healthy otherwise. Other secretly starchy veggies include carrots, peas, and corn. The next time you need a vegetable side or want to add something to a salad, reach for some bell peppers, broccoli, asparagus, or artichokes.

Lose the Juice

Fruit juice isn't as healthy as people once thought. It lacks the fiber of whole fruit, and even 100% fruit juice is loaded with sugar and carbs.

Cutting out fruit juice from your diet can eliminate a source of carbs you may not have even been watching out for.

Go with Protein for Breakfast

Even healthy breakfast cereals like granola and oatmeal are high in carbohydrates. But if you start your day with a protein, particularly eggs, you won't get off on the wrong foot. Eating protein early in the day also kick-starts your digestive system and helps you start burning fat when you exercise.

Cut the Crust

While pizza is an undeniably delicious indulgence, most pizza crusts are high in refined white flour, which is a major carbohydrate offender. If you can't resist eating pizza, opt for the thin crust variety rather than deep dish. You can still get your cheese and tomato sauce fix without ingesting as many carbohydrates.

Replace Your Rice

Rice, like pasta, is a carb-heavy starch that's omnipresent in many cuisines. But you don't have to give up on Chinese or Indian food entirely just because you're counting carbs. Try subbing in riced cauliflower. It's got a similar texture and absorbency, and when it's loaded up with curry or broccoli beef, you'll barely notice a difference.

Switch Your Chips

Potato chips are one of those snacks that it's really tough to let go of. If you're craving that crunch, try kale chips, which offer the same snackability with fewer carbs and a host of other health benefits. You can even make your own by tossing chopped up kale in olive oil, separating the leaves on a cooking sheet, and throwing them in the oven until they crisp up.

Wrap It Up

Sacrificing sandwiches and burgers is one of the toughest things about going low carb. But if you "think outside the bun," you can still enjoy many of the flavors you love, just low carb. The solution? Substitute lettuce wraps for the bun on your burger or the bread on your turkey sandwich. You'll drastically lower the carb content and still have something to grip.

Simple Tips and Exercise Plans to Lose Weight

There are several ways to lose weight fast and melt away your fat instantly. However, most of them leave you unsatisfied as one realizes that shortcuts to lose weight are not sustainable in the long run. Weight loss is a combination of a well-formulated diet plan and a rigorous exercise regime. If you are wondering how to lose weight here are a few simple tips for weight loss and exercise plans to lose weight and reduce those inches.

Water is your savior

Make sure to stay hydrated with water and other fluids throughout the day. One must drink at least 8 glasses of water a day to prevent all that bloating. A glass of water with lemon in it is recommended right after you wake up.

Fiber is key to a healthy gut

Food like vegetables are high in fiber, which prevent constipation and also helps one get a flat belly soon. It also helps in better digestion and improving your immune system in the long run.

Train your mind

Weight loss is about a good diet, rigorous exercise regime but most importantly about mental conviction. Before starting out on a weight loss journey, mentally make a note of why you are taking this step and keep this reason to keep you going and prevent you from catering to those cravings by binge eating.

Stay away from fad diets

The market today is flooded with diets like the GM diet, Atkins, Keto diet which all have very serious consequences to out bodies in the long run. Anything that comes fast, goes fast so remember to be patient and eat everything but in moderation.

Avoid food with high sugar content

Insulin is the fat storage hormone in our bodies and sugary foods like desserts release insulin. This instantly raises our blood sugar level in turn resulting in fat storage. Lowering insulin also works as a detox for the body allowing kidneys to expel any excess sodium or nitrates, which may cause bloating. It s important to completely cut out fizzy drinks which also cause gas.

Do not leave out a food group

Every year the weight loss industry makes one or the other food group the worst for the body. It is best to have all fats, carbs and proteins as part of our diet. Food rich in protein has been shown to boost ones metabolism and also reduces cravings

Eating Out? Make the Right Choices

Eating out is very common in today's world. One does not want to be the odd one out by always refusing to eat out with friends, family and colleagues in a bid to eat good home cooked meals and sticking to their health goals. Also, people are travelling more from what they used to once - whether it is for work or for leisure. However, it is possible to have a balanced and healthy lifestyle while still eating outside of home. All that is needed is making sound choices.

While eating food at a restaurant or at a food café or at a buffet, we may not know which food options are loaded with fat and calories. This becomes difficult for people on weight loss programs or those with clinical conditions. But, it does not mean that they do not eat out. Today healthier options are available at restaurants and food cafés and good choices can be made at buffets.

Just following the simple guidelines below will help you make healthy and guilt free food choices:

Be aware of overeating at a buffet

Check the entire buffet before you start filling your plate. Always start with a soup (non-creamy, broth based), fill the plate with veggies; opt for non-fried and less oily options. Instead of sugar sweetened beverages opt for plain water, buttermilk or jal jeera. Avoid butter / oil laden kulchas, puris, parathas, butter nan and ask for plain wheat rotis. Instead of desserts go for fresh cut fruit plate. Always wait for 5 to 10 minutes before going for a second helping.

Salad tips

Those opting for salads before the main course tend to eat fewer overall calories. However, avoid creamy cheese, honey based dressings, cheese, potatoes, bacon, fried noodles, croutons etc in salads as they are high in calories. Instead, squeeze a lemon or try rice vinegar or balsamic vinegar. If you want to order a dressing based salad ask for the dressing on the side as then the amount of dressing you put in the salad will be in your control. A salad with just some vegetables, corn, lean meat or beans could be a great filler. Stir fries can also be a great option instead of the salad to help you avoid eating more calories later.

Skip the fancy drinks

Both, alcoholic and non alcoholic drinks add to only calories in a meal. The margaritas, pina coladas and the other fancy drinks are laden with sugar. If a drink is must, a glass of wine or a simple martini can be an option. For those preferring a non alcoholic drink, buttermilk, jal jeera or a light lemonade can keep away the unwanted calories. However, plain water is always the best option.

Appetizers and Soups

Avoid fried or breaded appetizers, which are generally high in calories. Of course, you can also save calories by skipping the appetizer altogether. Steamed appetizers like momos, grilled chicken, dimsums, etc are good options. When choosing soups the best choices are broth-based or tomato-based soups. Cream soups, chowders and pureed soups can contain heavy cream or egg yolks.

Make your meals low in fat

When you go out at a restaurant to eat always check how the food is prepared. Check whether the food is broiled, poached, grilled, baked, or steamed as it tends to be lower in fat than foods that are fried. Limit foods that come with cream sauce or gravy. Avoid or have butter, sour cream, gravy, and sauces served on the side. This will allow you to control how much you eat as they are high in fat and calories. While ordering for burgers and sandwiches avoid ordering them with cheese, bacon, and other sweet sauces and opt for whole wheat or multigrain bread with added vegetables. With sandwich meals, choose water and fruit or plain yogurt if they're available, rather than sugary or carbonated drinks, chips, and fries. Choose seafood, chicken, or lean red meat rather than fatty or processed meats.

Add fruits, vegetables, and whole grains

At fast food restaurant ask if french fries can be replaced by fruit or salad. Order extra vegetables with pizza, sandwiches etc. Indian, Thai and Japanese restaurants have a lot of vegetarian options available. Always opt for brown rice, whole wheat pasta, whole wheat or multigrain bread and tortillas instead of white rice, pasta, or white bread.

Watch the portion sizes

At restaurants, since the dish ordered is usually sufficient for 2-3 people, split the dish with your partner instead of eating the entire portion yourself. If you are at a fast food restaurant, order the small sized meal instead of the large sized one. Let go of the fries and the carbonated beverages.

Be conscious of what you eat while travelling

At hotel breakfast buffets do not eat large portions. Have a healthy mix of foods rich in carbohydrates and proteins with some fresh fruits. Make healthier food choices at meal times. Always drink plenty of water during travel as that is one aspect often neglected. Pack healthy snack options like roasted makhanas, nuts like almonds, walnuts, pistachios, dried fruits like dates, anjeer, apricots, raisins etc to avoid unhealthy snacking. Instead of drinking carbonated beverages always check for the availability of coconut water, buttermilk etc. Fresh fruits are also a good option to keep yourself from indulging in fried and other unhealthy foods.

Keto Diet Myths

The ketogenic diet is currently trending as the best diet for weight loss to date. It's a high-fat, low-carbohydrate diet that produces ketones— the result of the breakdown of fats in the liver — to be used as energy.

With the keto diet showing up all over the news, in forums, magazines, and in conversations at the gym, there's a lot of things being said that are true, but a lot of things that aren't so true as well.

Keto is a high-fat, high-protein diet

Unlike other low-carb diets, such as the Atkin's Diet, the keto diet is not particularly high in protein. In fact, protein intake actually must be "moderate" while on the keto diet because this allows you to transition into ketosis and stay there. Too much protein in your diet will actually result in some of the protein being converted to glucose (or sugar) once consumed — and obviously this is counterproductive when it comes to keeping glucose levels very low.

So how much protein do you need? A standard recommendation for following the ketogenic diet is to get about 75 percent of daily calories from sources of fat (such as oils or fattier cuts of meat), 5 percent from carbohydrates, and 20 percent from protein (give or take a little depending on the individual). In contrast, high-protein, low-carb diets might entail getting 30–35 percent (or more) of daily calories from protein.

It's dangerous

It's dangerous. It's not dangerous if you're careful.

Just like with anything there are downsides, but the ketogenic diet isn't inherently dangerous.

Everyday Health lists the potential downsides, including: kidney stones, vitamin and mineral deficiencies, decreased bone mineral density, gastrointestinal distress, and an increased risk of higher cholesterol and heart disease.

Staying hydrated, easing into fasting if you choose to do so, and ensuring you know and hit your daily macros are essential to avoiding these potential downsides.

Keto is the same for men and women

Overall women are more sensitive to effects of dietary changes and weight loss compared to men. It's definitely possible for women to safely follow the keto diet, and to practice intermittent fasting if they choose, but they should do so more carefully. It's recommended that women focus on eating an alkaline diet in addition to a keto diet, meaning they include lots of non-starchy vegetables to make sure they obtain enough electrolytes and nutrients. The diet should ideally be approached in step-wise fashion, focusing on alkaline first before adding in fasting and the keto aspect.

Women should also reduce other sources of stress as much as possible and always listen to their bodies. Stress can cause hormonal changes that might make ketosis more difficult to withstand. If you're a women following the keto diet then always pay attention to how exercise impacts your energy and moods, how much sleep you get nightly, the amount of sunlight exposure you get, your alcohol and caffeine intake, and the level of environmental toxicity you're exposed to. Make adjustments as needed if you feel run down or overwhelmed by the diet, since pushing yourself too hard may backfire.

Keto is a weight loss diet only

No doubt about it, the ketogenic diet can definitely help many people with weight loss and fat burning. But if losing weight is not one of your goals, this doesn't mean you can't follow the keto diet and maintain or even gain weight.

Can you gain weight on the keto diet? It's certainly possible, especially if you don't follow the diet correctly and aren't actually in ketosis.

There's some controversy surrounding the topic of weight loss due to very high-fat, low-carb diets: some people believe that weight loss is due to decreasing calorie intake, while others believe it's due to the hormonal effects that the diet has. Still, most experts will agree that despite the type of diet someone follows, if calorie intake exceeds someone's needs then weight loss can still occur, no matter where the calories come from.

The bottom line? If you eat more calories consistently than you actually need, even if the calories are from fat or protein sources, then you may start to see the scale creep up.

Maybe you're wondering, "If someone is not looking to lose weight, why would they still follow the keto diet"? The benefits of the ketogenic diet extend far beyond weight loss — they also include regulating hormone production, helping to normalize blood sugar, improving cognitive functioning, improving digestive health, and potentially even reducing the risk for certain diseases and disorders like diabetes or heart disease.

Going keto means zero alcohol consumption

Going keto means zero alcohol consumption. Some liquors, beers, and wines are OK on Keto.

Beer and wine are generally carbohydrate-heavy, but there are still options should you choose to continue drinking alcohol while going keto. Most liquors, some light beers, and dry wines are low to no carb, which is keto friendly.

Alcohol isn't totally out of the question, but you do have to be a bit more conscious of what you choose, and careful when drinking and going keto. Keep in mind that your alcohol tolerance will likely be lower while eating ketogenic.

Everyone gets the keto flu

Every person reacts to the ketogenic diet somewhat differently, so it's hard to say what type of side effects you might experience, how severe they will be, and for how long they will last. Some people transition into ketosis smoothly, while others might deal with more fatigue, brain-fog, digestive issues and sleep-related problems for several weeks (this phase has been nicknamed "the keto flu").

While these side effects might be uncomfortable, it's common for them to go away within a couple weeks, so try to be patient. You can reduce the changes that you'll experience side effects by consuming enough water, salt, fiber and electrolytes (like potassium or magnesium) from vegetables.

You will always be low energy on keto

Many find that after they adjust to being in ketosis their energy and concentration actually increases. Initially your energy might be lower than normal, but it's likely that this will change. Ketones do a great job of providing the brain with a steady fuel-source, so it's common to experience more mental clarity, increased focus and more upbeat moods once you get going on the keto diet.

It's true that the diet is not just butter and coconut oil, but it's still quite high in saturated fat. A lack of boredom doesn't imply that it's a health-promoting plan either.

You said it yourself: You take a supplement to protect yourself from deficiencies, including (but not limited to) iron and zinc. You're also at risk for missing potassium, magnesium, folic acid, and beta carotene. Know that the FDA doesn't oversee supplements, so you may not be getting exactly what you pay for. Plus, certain nutrients consumed as supplements can also have a pro-oxidant effect, meaning they do more harm than good. The end result: Increased risk of chronic disease, including heart disease and some cancers.

You can't exercise on keto

Exercise is something that's beneficial for just about everybody, including those on the keto diet. Initially you might feel less energized during your workouts, but this should dissipate as your body adjusts. Even in the midst of high-intensity workouts, the ketogenic diet doesn't seem to cause any decline in performance.

In order to support your workouts, make sure you consume enough calories in general and plenty of fat. Also give yourself ample time for recovery between tougher workouts.

If you're really struggling with being active and recovering while on the diet then consider upping your carbs a bit and trying more of a "modified ketogenic diet" that is more flexible. If you plan on fasting while following the keto diet, then save your tough, high-intensity workouts for days/times of the day when you're more fueled.

Fasting is a requirement of the ketogenic diet

It's not a requirement; you do not have to fast to go keto. Too, it's typically not recommended that you incorporate fasting into the keto diet until you've eased into the process, such as lowering your carb intake slowly or going alkaline first.

However, intermittent fasting while going keto does have many benefits. It can accelerate weight loss, detoxification, and help control hunger and cravings.

Tips to Get Into Ketosis

Ketosis is a normal metabolic process that provides several health benefits.

During ketosis, your body converts fat into compounds known as ketones and begins using them as its main source of energy.

Studies have found that diets that promote ketosis are highly beneficial for weight loss, due in part to their appetite-suppressing effects.

Emerging research suggests that ketosis may also be helpful for type 2 diabetes and neurological disorders, among other conditions.

That being said, achieving a state of ketosis can take some work and planning. It's not just as simple as cutting carbs.

Here are effective tips to get into ketosis.

Know What You Should Focus On

Do calories matter on keto? What exactly should you eat? Why does the keto diet work so well?

Depending on who you ask, you may get a completely different answer. Even some research papers will propose one hypothesis while other data clearly suggests that it's not true (like the carbohydrate-insulin hypothesis for obesity).

With all of the contradicting beliefs in the keto diet world, it is hard to know what is actually true — and without the truth how are you supposed to know what to do if things don't go as you initially hoped?

Do you focus on limiting carbs more? What about exercising? Should you intermittent fast?

After digging through the research, It becomes clear that people lose weight on keto because of one thing — the fact that keto dieters tend to eat much fewer calories than they did before without noticing.

It doesn't matter how much you restrict your carbs and how many grams of fat you eat. The key to burning off your own fat is being in a calorie deficit.

If you can find a diet that allows you to eat fewer calories than before without battling against cravings and hunger (like keto dieting does for most people), then you've found one of the most sustainable ways to lose weight.

The best way to create a diet like this is by following these two principles:

- Eating mostly protein-dense and fiber-rich foods because of how satiating they are.
- Eliminating all calorically-dense processed foods from your diet because of how easy it is to binge on them.

The primary reason why the keto diet is so effective for weight loss is that it follows these two principles better than almost every other popular diet. As a result, people who are following the keto diet feel more satisfied than ever before on fewer calories and start burning off excess body fat.

Minimize Your Carb Consumption

Eating a very low-carb diet is by far the most important factor in achieving ketosis.

Normally, your cells use glucose, or sugar, as their main source of fuel. However, most of your cells can also use other fuel sources. This includes fatty acids, as well as ketones, which are also known as ketone bodies.

Your body stores glucose in your liver and muscles in the form of glycogen.

When carb intake is very low, glycogen stores are reduced and levels of the hormone insulin decline. This allows fatty acids to be released from fat stores in your body.

Your liver converts some of these fatty acids into the ketone bodies acetone, acetoacetate and beta-hydroxybutyrate. These ketones can be used as fuel by portions of the brain.

The level of carb restriction needed to induce ketosis is somewhat individualized. Some people need to limit net carbs (total carbs minus fiber) to 20 grams per day, while others can achieve ketosis while eating twice this amount or more.

For this reason, the Atkins diet specifies that carbs be restricted to 20 or fewer grams per day for two weeks to guarantee that ketosis is achieved.

After this point, small amounts of carbs can be added back to your diet very gradually, as long as ketosis is maintained.

In a one-week study, overweight people with type 2 diabetes who limited carb intake to 21 or fewer grams per day experienced daily urinary ketone excretion levels that were 27 times higher than their baseline levels.

In another study, adults with type 2 diabetes were allowed 20–50 grams of digestible carbs per day, depending on the number of grams that allowed them to maintain blood ketone levels within a target range of 0.5–3.0 mmol/L.

These carb and ketone ranges are advised for people who want to get into ketosis to promote weight loss, control blood sugar levels or reduce heart disease risk factors.

In contrast, therapeutic ketogenic diets used for epilepsy or as experimental cancer therapy often restrict carbs to fewer than 5% of calories or fewer than 15 grams per day to further drive up ketone levels.

However, anyone using the diet for therapeutic purposes should only do so under the supervision of a medical professional.

Increase Your Healthy Fat Intake

Consuming plenty of healthy fat can boost your ketone levels and help you reach ketosis.

Indeed, a very low-carb ketogenic diet not only minimizes carbs, but is also high in fat.

Ketogenic diets for weight loss, metabolic health and exercise performance usually provide between 60–80% of calories from fat.

The classic ketogenic diet used for epilepsy is even higher in fat, with typically 85–90% of calories from fat.

However, extremely high fat intake doesn't necessarily translate into higher ketone levels.

A three-week study of 11 healthy people compared the effects of fasting with different amounts of fat intake on breath ketone levels.

Overall, ketone levels were found to be similar in people consuming 79% or 90% of calories from fat.

Furthermore, because fat makes up such a large percentage of a ketogenic diet, it's important to choose high-quality sources.

Good fats include olive oil, avocado oil, coconut oil, butter, lard and tallow. In addition, there are many healthy, high-fat foods that are also very low in carbs.

However, if your goal is weight loss, it's important to make sure you're not consuming too many calories in total, as this can cause your weight loss to stall.

Only Consume Keto Foods and Ingredients

Keto foods are foods and ingredients that are very low in carbs. What "very low in carbs" means exactly will depend on your daily carb limit. For example, we recommend keeping total carbs below 35g and net carbs below 25g (ideally, below 20g) so that you can reap the benefits of eating highly satiating foods and ketosis. (To figure out your net carb consumption, simply subtract total fiber intake from total carbs.)

To have such a small amount of carbs, you must be vigilant about your food choices. You may find that many of your favorite foods will put you near your carbohydrate limit for the day with just one serving. Even healthier foods like fruits and vegetables are packed with sugar and carbs, but don't get discouraged — there is plenty of delicious food you can eat on the ketogenic diet.

Do Eat

- Meats – fish, beef, lamb, poultry, eggs, etc.
- Low carb vegetables – spinach, kale, broccoli, cauliflower, and other keto-friendly vegetables >

- High fat dairy – hard cheeses, high fat cream, butter, etc.
- Nuts and seeds – macadamias, walnuts, sunflower seeds, etc.
- Avocado and berries – raspberries, blackberries, and other low glycemic impact berries
- Sweeteners – stevia, erythritol, monk fruit, and other low-carb sweeteners >
- Other fats – coconut oil, high-fat salad dressing, saturated fats, etc.

Do Not Eat

- Tubers – potato, yams, etc.
- Fruit – apples, bananas, oranges, etc.
- Sugar – honey, agave, maple syrup, etc.
- Grains – wheat, corn, rice, cereal, etc.

Include Coconut Oil in Your Diet

Eating coconut oil can help you get into ketosis.

It contains fats called medium-chain triglycerides (MCTs).

Unlike most fats, MCTs are rapidly absorbed and taken directly to the liver, where they can be used immediately for energy or converted into ketones.

In fact, it's been suggested that consuming coconut oil may be one of the best ways to increase ketone levels in people with Alzheimer's disease and other nervous system disorders.

Although coconut oil contains four types of MCTs, 50% of its fat comes from the kind known as lauric acid.

Some research suggests that fat sources with a higher percentage of lauric acid may produce a more sustained level of ketosis. This is because it's metabolized more gradually than other MCTs.

MCTs have been used to induce ketosis in epileptic children without restricting carbs as drastically as the classic ketogenic diet.

In fact, several studies have found that a high-MCT diet containing 20% of calories from carbs produces effects similar to the classic ketogenic diet, which provides fewer than 5% of calories from carbs.

When adding coconut oil to your diet, it's a good idea to do so slowly to minimize digestive side effects like stomach cramping or diarrhea.

Start with one teaspoon per day and work up to two to three tablespoons daily over the course of a week.

Track Your Macros

One of the best ways to track what you are eating is by using a calorie tracking app and a scale. By using both, you will be much more accurate in knowing what you are consuming and have all the info you need to start losing weight consistently again.

When it comes to tracking calories, I prefer to use MyFitnessPal (for general macro tracking) and Cronometer (for more specific macro and micronutrient tracking). If you'd like to get started with tracking your calories using these apps, check out our guide on the topic — It has everything you need to know so that you can set up MyFitnessPal and Cronometer for your specific macronutrient needs.

To find out what your calorie and macronutrient needs are, plug your info into our keto calculator. It will tell you exactly how many calories and grams of fat, protein, and carbs you need to eat on a daily basis to get the results you want.

Another way to increase the accuracy of your calorie tracking is by using a food scale. Most people measure the amount of food they eat by guesstimating – which typically causes you to eat more calories than you intend.

There are certain things you should look for when buying a scale, and most importantly include:

- *Having a conversion button.* Most calorie tracking apps and websites use a mixture of units. Having a conversion button on your scale can make it much easier for you to measure your food. A gram to ounce and ounce to gram conversion button is the one that I most commonly use.
- *Automatic Shutoff.* Make sure you research the scale you are buying. If the scales have an automatic shutoff, it can be troublesome to properly measure your food. Try to find scales that allow you to program the automatic shutoff or require you to manually turn it off.

- *Tare Function.* Being able to place bowls, plates, and utensils on your scale makes it a lot easier to weight things out. Make sure that your scale has a tare option, which will allow you to place an item on the scale and revert back to 0.
- *Removable Plate.* Cleaning scales can be a huge hassle when dealing with messy foods. Double check that the scale you are buying has a removable plate for easy cleaning.

Keto Diet Recipes

1 Ham & Broccoli Frittata

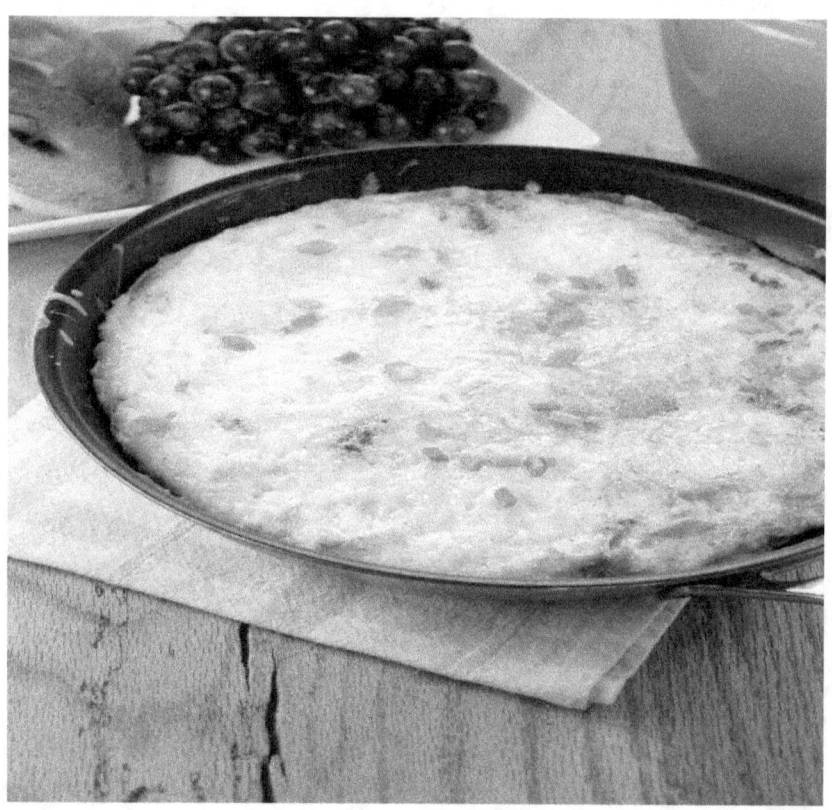

With just five ingredients, this cheesy frittata is a breeze to make. It's sure to become a new family favorite.

Prep/Cook Time: 30 min.
4 servings

Ingredients

- 6 large eggs
- 1/4 teaspoon pepper
- Dash salt
- 1-1/4 cups shredded Swiss cheese, divided
- 1 cup cubed fully cooked ham
- 1 tablespoon butter
- 1 cup chopped fresh broccoli

Instructions

- Preheat broiler. In a bowl, whisk eggs, pepper and salt. Stir in 1 cup cheese and ham.
- In a 10-in. ovenproof skillet, heat butter over medium-high heat. Add broccoli; cook and stir until tender. Reduce heat to low; pour in egg mixture. Cook, covered, 4-6 minutes or until nearly set. Sprinkle with remaining cheese.
- Broil 3-4 in. from heat 2-3 minutes or until eggs are completely set. Let stand 5 minutes. Cut into wedges.

Nutrition Info

- 1 wedge: 321 calories
- 23g fat (11g saturated fat)
- 374mg cholesterol
- 665mg sodium
- 4g carbohydrate (2g sugars, 1g fiber)
- 26g protein.

2 Oven Denver Omelet

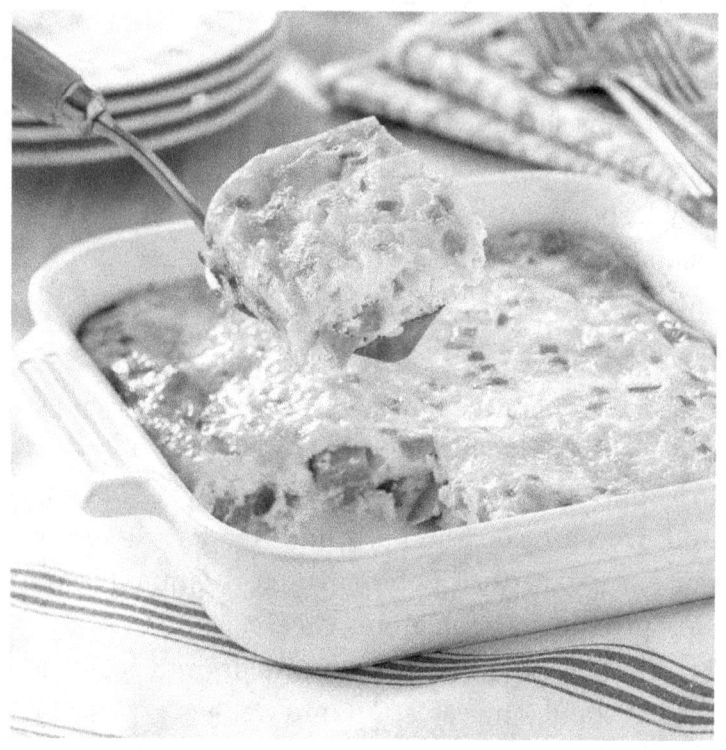

Prep/Cook Time: 30 min.

6 servings

Ingredients

- 8 large eggs
- 1/2 cup half-and-half cream
- 1 cup shredded cheddar cheese
- 1 cup finely chopped fully cooked ham
- 1/4 cup finely chopped green pepper
- 1/4 cup finely chopped onion

Instructions

- In a large bowl, whisk eggs and cream. Stir in the cheese, ham, green pepper and onion. Pour into a greased 9-in. square baking dish.
- Bake at 400° for 25 minutes or until golden brown.

Nutrition Info

1 piece: 235 calories	16g fat (8g saturated fat)
326mg cholesterol	506mg sodium
4g carbohydrate	17g protein.

3 Savory Apple-Chicken Sausage

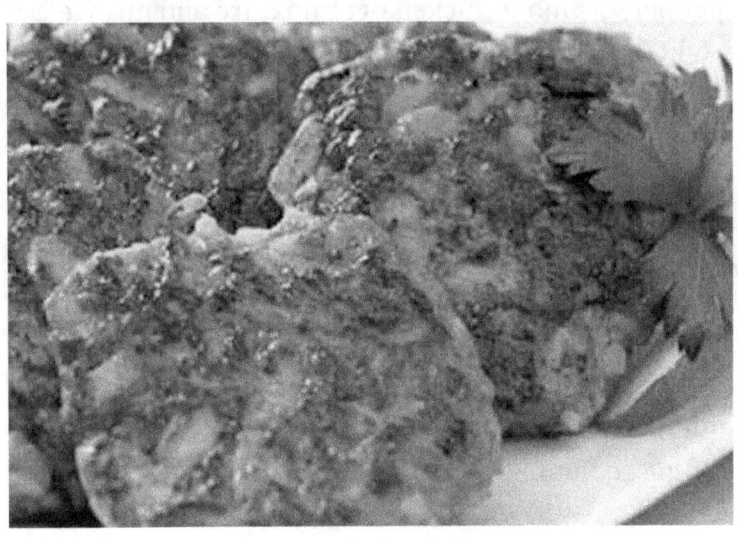

These easy, healthy sausages taste great, and they make an elegant brunch dish. The recipe is also very versatile. It can be doubled or tripled for a crowd, and the sausage freezes well either cooked or raw.

Prep/Cook Time: 25 min.
Servings: 8 patties

Ingredients

- 1 large tart apple, peeled and diced
- 2 teaspoons poultry seasoning
- 1 teaspoon salt
- 1/4 teaspoon pepper
- 1 pound ground chicken

Instructions

- In a large bowl, combine the apple, poultry seasoning, salt and pepper. Crumble chicken over mixture and mix well. Shape into eight 3-in. patties.
- In a large, greased cast-iron or other heavy skillet, cook patties over medium heat until no longer pink, 5-6 minutes on each side. Drain if necessary.

Nutrition Info

1 sausage patty: 92 calories
5g fat (1g saturated fat)
38mg cholesterol
328mg sodium
4g carbohydrate (3g sugars, 1g fiber)
9g protein.

4 Zucchini Frittata

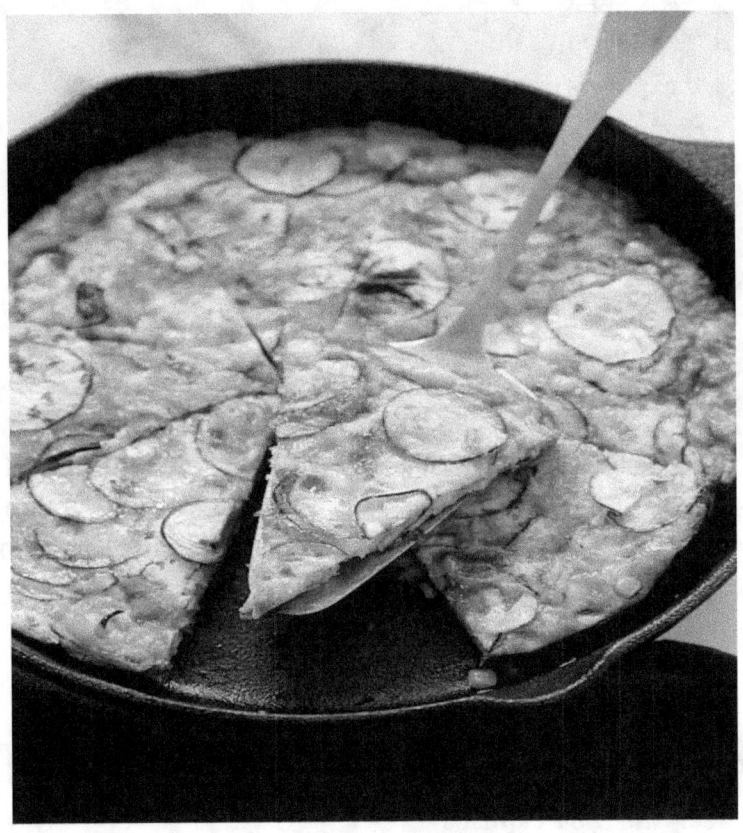

When we travel by car, I make the frittata the night before, stuff it into pita bread in the morning and microwave for a minute or two before I wrap them in a towel so down the road we enjoy a still-warm breakfast!

Prep/Cook Time: 20 min.
2 servings

Ingredients

- 3 large eggs
- 1/4 teaspoon salt
- 1 teaspoon canola oil
- 1/2 cup chopped onion
- 1 cup coarsely shredded zucchini
- 1/2 cup shredded Swiss cheese
- Coarsely ground pepper, optional

Instructions

- Preheat oven to 350°. Whisk together eggs and salt.
- In an 8-in. ovenproof skillet coated with cooking spray, heat oil over medium heat; saute onion and zucchini until onion is crisp-tender. Pour in egg mixture; cook until almost set, 5-6 minutes. Sprinkle with cheese.
- Bake, uncovered, until cheese is melted, 4-5 minutes. If desired, sprinkle with pepper.

Nutrition Info

1 serving: 261 calories

18g fat (8g saturated fat)

304mg cholesterol

459mg sodium

7g carbohydrate (3g sugars, 1g fiber)

18g protein.

5 Mini Spinach Frittatas

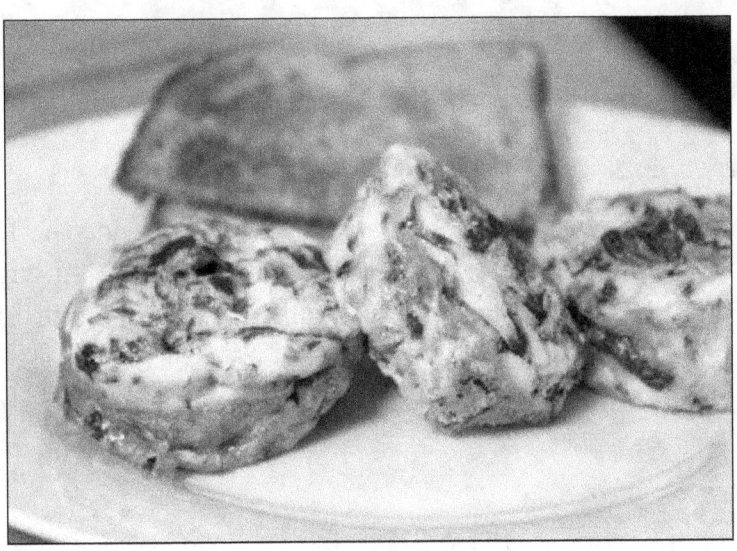

People can't get enough of these pop-in-your-mouth mini frittatas. They're a cinch to make, freeze well and the recipe easily doubles for a crowd.

Prep/Cook Time: 30 min.
2 dozen

Ingredients
- 1 cup whole-milk ricotta cheese
- 3/4 cup grated Parmesan cheese
- 2/3 cup chopped fresh mushrooms
- 1 package (10 ounces) frozen chopped spinach, thawed and squeezed dry
- 1 large egg

- 1/2 teaspoon dried oregano
- 1/4 teaspoon salt
- 1/4 teaspoon pepper
- 24 slices pepperoni

Instructions

- Preheat oven to 375°. In a small bowl, combine the first eight ingredients. Place a pepperoni slice in each of 24 greased mini-muffin cups; fill three-fourths full with cheese mixture.
- Bake 20-25 minutes or until completely set. Carefully run a knife around sides of muffin cups to loosen frittatas. Serve warm.

Nutrition Info

1 mini frittata: 128 calories

9g fat (5g saturated fat)

50mg cholesterol

396mg sodium

4g carbohydrate (2g sugars, 1g fiber)

10g protein.

6 Frittata Florentine

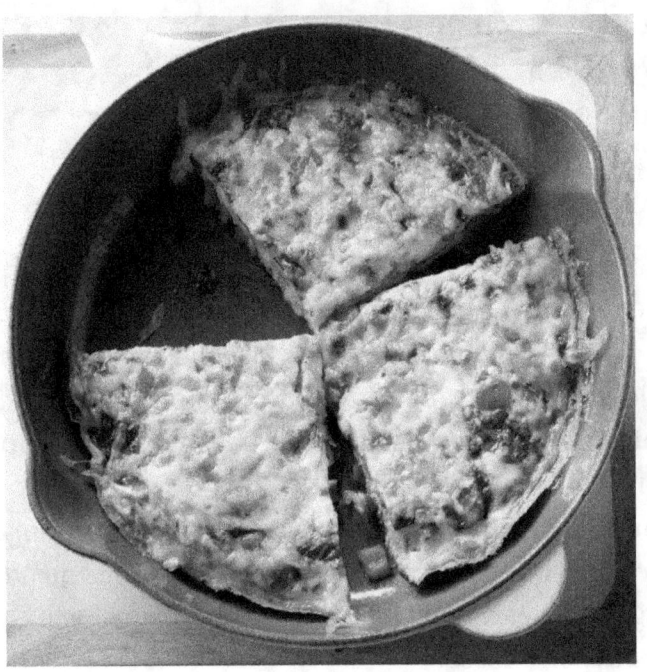

Prep/Cook Time: 30 min.

4 servings

Ingredients

- 6 large egg whites
- 3 large eggs
- 1/2 teaspoon dried oregano
- 1/4 teaspoon garlic powder
- 1/4 teaspoon salt
- 1/4 teaspoon pepper
- 1 tablespoon olive oil

- 1 small onion, finely chopped
- 1/4 cup finely chopped sweet red pepper
- 2 turkey bacon strips, chopped
- 1 cup fresh baby spinach
- 3 tablespoons thinly sliced fresh basil leaves
- 1/2 cup shredded part-skim mozzarella cheese

Instructions

- Preheat broiler. In a small bowl, whisk the first six ingredients.
- In an 8-in. ovenproof skillet, heat oil over medium-high heat. Add onion, red pepper and bacon; cook and stir 4-5 minutes or until onion is tender. Reduce heat to medium-low; top with spinach.
- Pour in egg mixture. As eggs set, push cooked portions toward the center, letting uncooked eggs flow underneath; cook until eggs are nearly thickened. Remove from heat; sprinkle with basil, then cheese.
- Broil 3-4 in. from heat 2-3 minutes or until eggs are completely set. Let stand 5 minutes. Cut into wedges.

Tip

Want to be super healthy? Substitute 6 egg whites for the 3 whole eggs listed in the ingredients, you'll be using a total of 12 egg whites to complete the recipe.

Nutrition Info

1 slice: 176 calories
174mg cholesterol
4g carbohydrate

11g fat (4g saturated fat)
451mg sodium
15g protein.

7 Broccoli and Cauliflower Salad with Capers in Lemon Vinaigrette

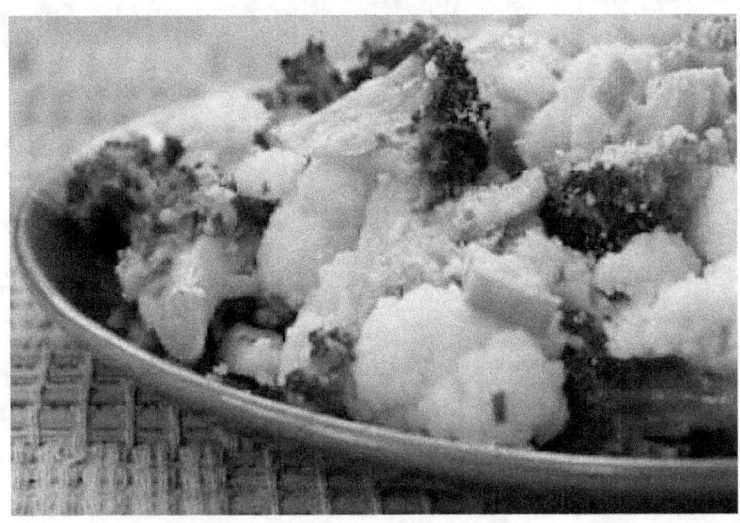

A quick and easy salad, perfect for the warmer weather or if you're looking for a different way to make broccoli. This lemon vinaigrette makes any vegetable taste delicious.

Total Time: 20 mins
Servings 6 servings

Ingredients
- 1 13 oz head broccoli
- 1 13 oz head cauliflower
- 2 tbsp capers

For the Vinaigrette:

- Juice from 1/2 lemon, 2 tbsp
- 3 tbsp extra virgin olive oil
- 1 clove garlic, crushed
- 1 small shallot, minced
- Salt and pepper

Instructions

- In a small bowl, whisk the lemon juice, olive oil, garlic, shallot, salt and pepper.
- Cut the broccoli and cauliflower into bite size florets. Using a steamer, steam the vegetables for about 5 minutes. Remove the vegetables, rinse under cold water to stop them from cooking, drain and place in a large bowl.
- Toss with the vinaigrette and serve.

Nutrition Info

Serving: 1/6th
Calories: 97kcal
Carbohydrates: 7.6g
Protein: 3.2g
Fat: 7g

8 Tuna Salad Wraps

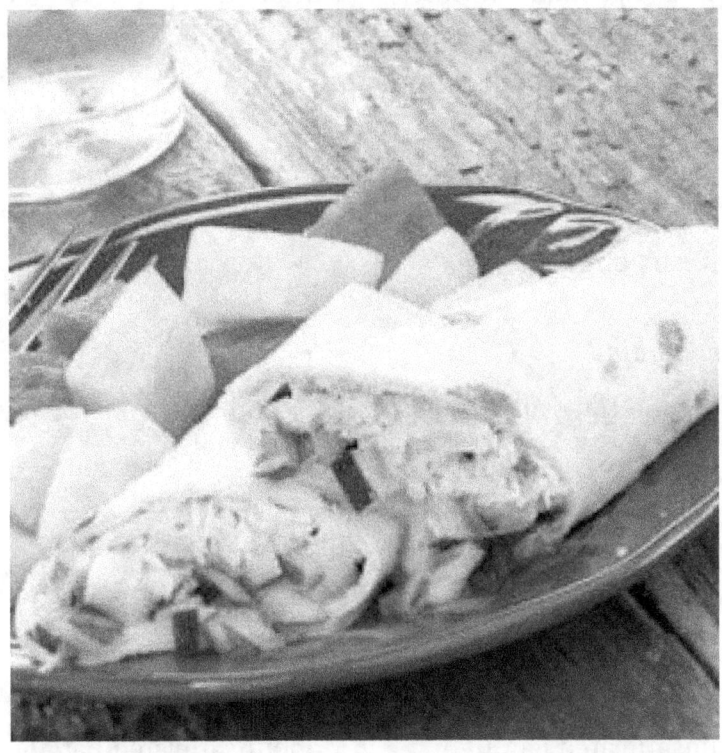

This is an easy, light lunch recipe, or appetizer, using canned tuna with chopped red onion and a little red wine vinegar and added broccoli and celery, served on spinach leaves.

Prep Time: 10 mins
Total Time: 10 mins
Servings 2 servings

Ingredients

- 1 can light tuna in water, 4 oz drained
- 1/4 cup chopped celery
- 1/4 cup chopped red onion
- 1/4 cup broccoli florets
- 2 tbsp Hellmann's light mayonnaise, regular for Keto
- 1 tsp red wine vinegar
- fresh pepper

Instructions

Drain tuna. Mix all the ingredients and serve in freshly washed spinach leaves.

Nutrition Info

Serving: 2servings

Calories: 160kcal

Carbohydrates: 4.5g

Protein: 22g

Fat: 6g

Saturated Fat: 1g

Polyunsaturated Fat: 0g

Monounsaturated Fat: 0g

Trans Fat: 0g

Cholesterol: 30mg

Sodium: 415mg

Potassium: 0mg

Fiber: 1g, Sugar: 1g

9 Roasted Spaghetti Squash

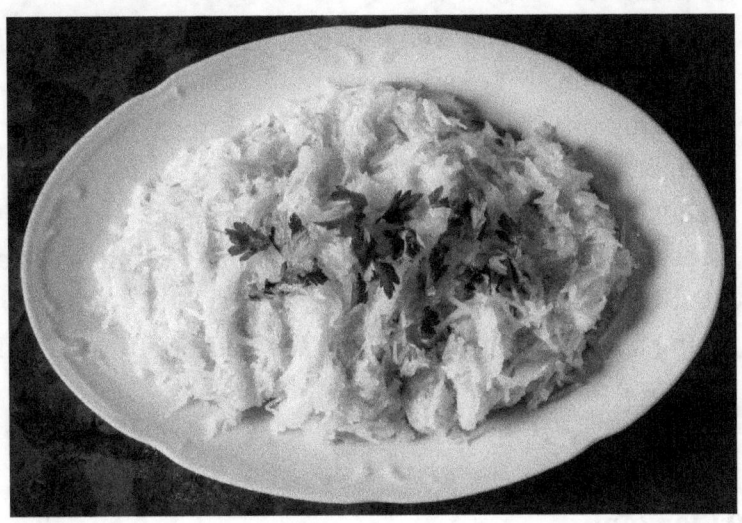

Spaghetti squash is so versatile and easy to make! Enjoy it with salt and pepper as a side dish, drizzle it with butter and grated cheese, or top it with tomato sauce to replace your favorite spaghetti dish. Here is a basic recipe for roasted spaghetti squash.

Total Time: 1 hr 15 mins
Servings 6 servings

Ingredients
- 1 large ripe spaghetti squash
- salt and fresh pepper

Instructions

- Preheat oven to 350°.
- Cut the squash in half lengthwise, scoop out the seeds and fibers with a spoon.
- Place on a baking sheet, cut side up and sprinkle with salt and pepper.
- Bake at 350° about an hour or until the skin gives easily under pressure and the inside is tender. Remove from oven and let it cool 10 minutes.
- Using a fork, scrape out the squash flesh a little at a time. It will separate into spaghetti-like strands.
- Place in a serving dish and serve hot.

Nutrition Info

Serving: 1cup
Calories: 42kcal
Carbohydrates: 10g
Protein: 1g
Fat: 0.4g
Polyunsaturated Fat: 0g
Monounsaturated Fat: 0g
Trans Fat: 0g
Sodium: 28mg

10 Spinach Feta Frittata

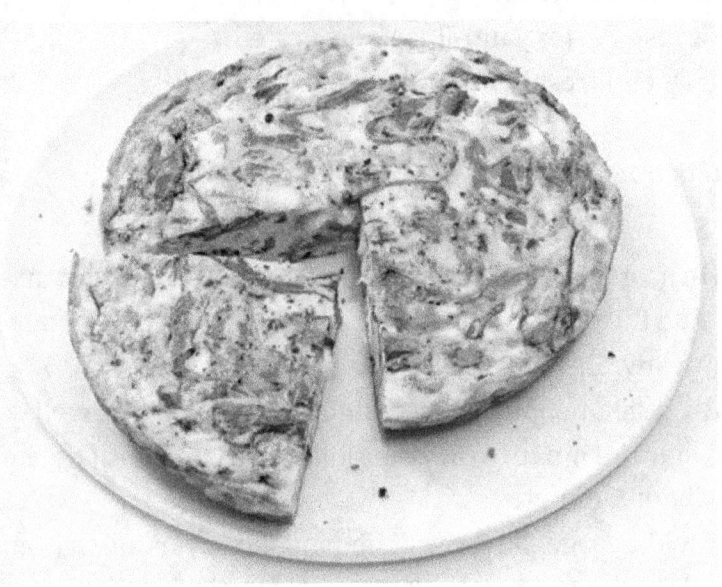

Spinach, scallions, feta and eggs make a fabulous, light breakfast frittata or for a low carb lunch serve this frittata with a Greek salad on the side.

Total Time: 25 mins
Servings 4 servings

Ingredients

- 2 whole eggs
- 8 large egg whites
- 1 tsp olive oil
- 1/2 red onion, finely chopped
- 3 scallions, chopped

- 10 oz frozen chopped spinach, thawed
- 2 oz crumbled feta
- 2 tbsp Parmigiano-Reggiano, grated
- salt and freshly ground pepper

Instructions

- Squeeze all water from spinach.
- In a 9 inch non-stick sauté pan, heat olive oil over medium heat.
- Add the onion and scallions and cook until soft, about 4 minutes.
- Meanwhile in a medium bowl, beat the eggs.
- Add salt, pepper, cheeses and spinach and mix well.
- Pour the mixture into the skillet and cook until the bottom sets, about 5 minutes.
- Hold a large plate over the pan and invert the frittata onto the plate, then slide it back into the pan.
- Cook about 5 minutes longer. Serve hot.

Nutrition Info

Serving: 1/4 of frittata
Calories: 141kcal
Carbohydrates: 5.5g
Protein: 15.2g
Fat: 6.8g
Saturated Fat: 3g

11 String Beans with Garlic and Oil

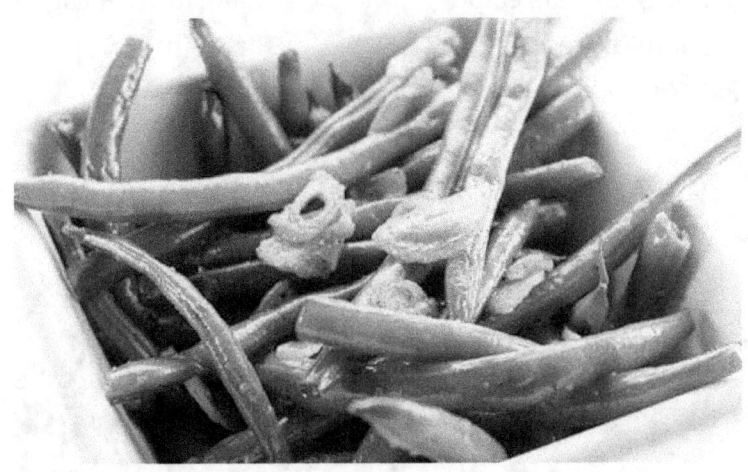

Total Time: 15 mins

Servings 4 servings

Ingredients

- 1 lb fresh string beans, washed, ends trimmed
- 2 tbsp extra virgin olive oil
- 4 cloves garlic, sliced thin
- salt and fresh pepper

Instructions

- Bring a large saucepan filled with 1 inch of water to a boil.
- Lower a steamer basket filled with the green beans into it, tightly cover the pan, and steam for 4-5 minutes (don't overcook), until the beans are tender crisp. Drain.
- In a saute pan heat olive oil. Add garlic and cook until golden.
- Add string beans, salt and fresh pepper to taste and toss well.

Nutrition Info

Serving: 1/4 of recipe

Calories: 99kcal

Carbohydrates: 9g

Protein: 2g

Fat: 7g

12 Baked Garlic Lemon Tilapia

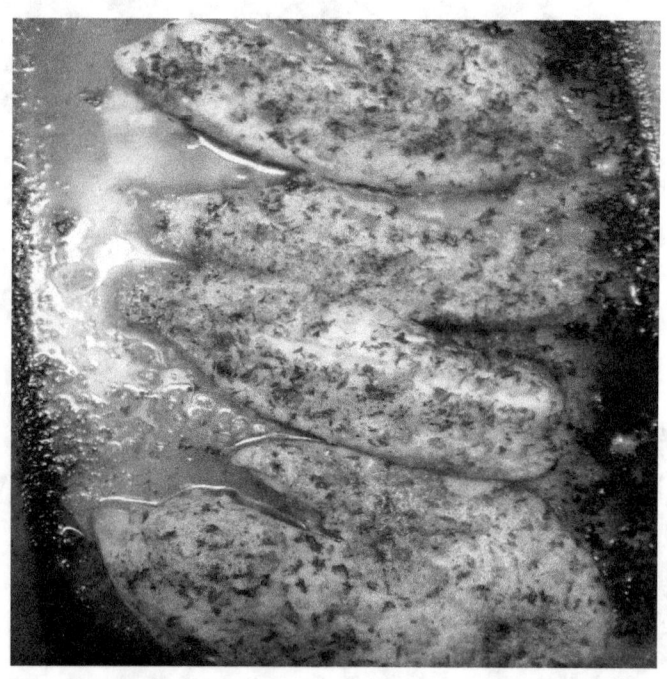

Classic sauce of butter, lemon and fresh parsley goes perfect with any fish. I try to eat fish twice a week. For a quick healthy dinner on a busy weeknight, this is simple and delicious.

Total Time: 30 mins

Servings 6 servings

Ingredients

- 6 6 oz each tilapia filets
- 4 cloves garlic, crushed
- 2 tbsp butter
- 2 tbsp fresh lemon juice
- 4 tsp fresh parsley
- salt and pepper
- cooking spray

Instructions

- Preheat oven to 400°.
- Melt butter on a low flame in a small sauce pan. Add garlic and saute on low for about 1 minute. Add the lemon juice and shut off flame.
- Spray the bottom of a baking dish lightly with cooking spray.
- Place the fish on top and season with salt and pepper. Pour the lemon butter mixture on the fish and top with fresh parsley.
- Bake at 400° until cooked, about 15 minutes.

Nutrition Info

Serving: 1piece fish

Calories: 199.5kcal

Carbohydrates: 1g

Protein: 33.5g

Fat: 7g

Polyunsaturated Fat: 0g

Monounsaturated Fat: 0g

Trans Fat: 0g

Sodium: 29mg

Potassium: 0mg

13 Asparagus-Mushroom Frittata

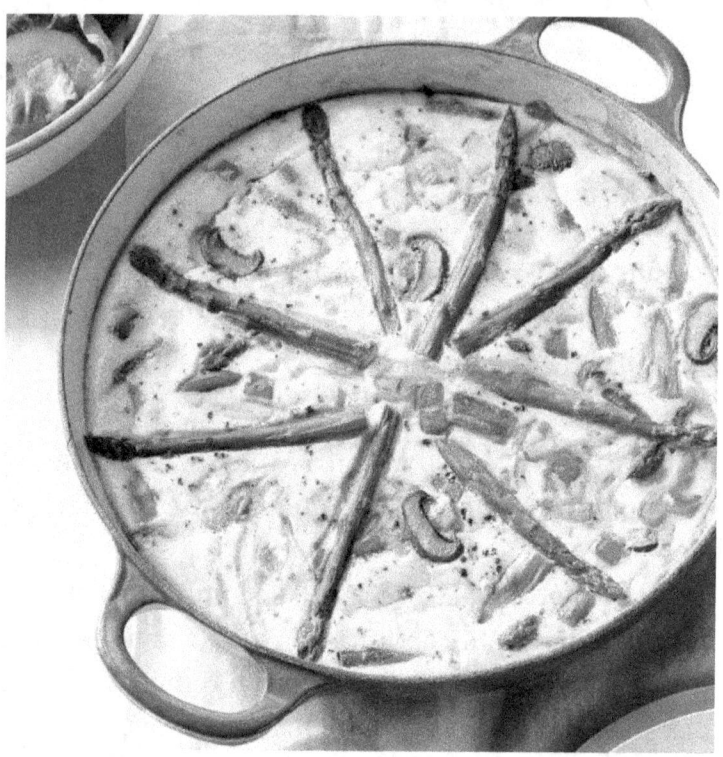

Prep: 25 min. Bake: 20 min.
8 servings

Ingredients

- 8 large eggs
- 1/2 cup whole-milk ricotta cheese
- 2 tablespoons lemon juice
- 1/2 teaspoon salt
- 1/4 teaspoon pepper

- 1 tablespoon olive oil
- 1 package (8 ounces) frozen asparagus spears, thawed
- 1 large onion, halved and thinly sliced
- 1/2 cup finely chopped sweet red or green pepper
- 1/4 cup sliced baby portobello mushrooms

Instructions

- Preheat oven to 350°. In a large bowl, whisk eggs, ricotta cheese, lemon juice, salt and pepper. In a 10-in. ovenproof skillet, heat oil over medium heat. Add asparagus, onion, red pepper and mushrooms; cook and stir 6-8 minutes or until onion and pepper are tender.
- Remove from heat; remove asparagus from skillet. Reserve eight spears; cut remaining asparagus into 2-in. pieces. Return cut asparagus to skillet; stir in egg mixture. Arrange reserved asparagus spears over eggs to resemble spokes of a wheel.
- Bake, uncovered, 20-25 minutes or until eggs are completely set. Let stand 5 minutes. Cut into wedges.

Nutrition Info

1 wedge: 130 calories
8g fat (3g saturated fat)
192mg cholesterol
240mg sodium
5g carbohydrate (3g sugars, 1g fiber)
9g protein.

14 Lighter Chicken Salad

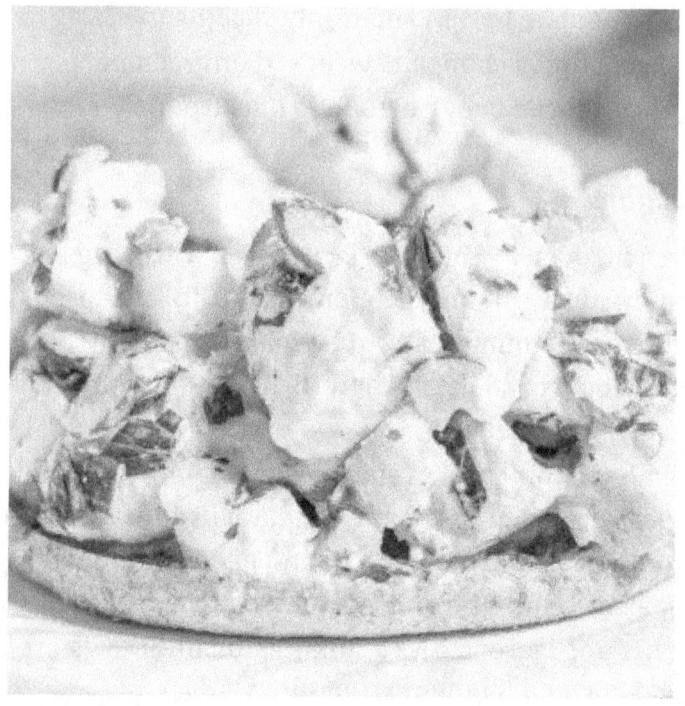

This lightened Classic chicken salad made from scratch uses far less mayonnaise that most recipes call for. It comes out tender and delicious, perfect on a bagel, served over lettuce or in a wrap.

Prep Time: 5 mins
Cook Time: 20 mins
Total Time: 25 mins
Servings 3 servings

Ingredients

- 2 pieces 1 lb boneless, skinless chicken breasts
- 1 chicken bouillon
- 1/4 onion, chopped
- 2 tbsp parsley chopped
- 2 celery stalks, finely chopped
- 3 tbsp Hellmann's Lite Mayonnaise, regular for Keto

Instructions

- In a medium sauce pan, place chicken, half the celery, half the onion, parsley and cover with water.
- Add bullion and cook on medium flame, covered for about 15-20 minutes, until chicken is cooked through.
- Once cooked, remove chicken and let cool. Reserve chicken broth.
- Cut chicken into small pieces and place in a bowl. Add onions, celery and mayonnaise, 1/8 cup reserved chicken broth and mix well. If looks dry add 1/8 cup more.
- Serve on a bed of lettuce, in a lettuce wrap or on your favorite bread.

Nutrition Info

Serving: 1/3
Carbohydrates: 4g
Fat: 5.5g
Monounsaturated Fat: 0g
Sodium: 664.5mg
Fiber: 1g

Calories: 169.5kcal
Protein: 25.5g
Polyunsaturated Fat: 0g
Trans Fat: 0g
Potassium: 0mg
Sugar: 0g

15 Asparagus with Dijon Vinaigrette

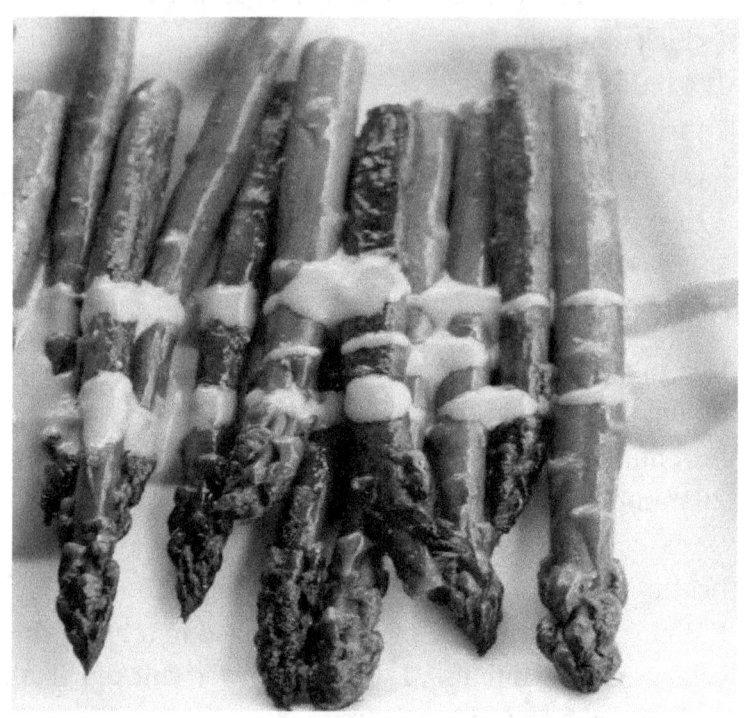

A simple asparagus side dish that really celebrates Spring. Serve it cold or room temperature, leftovers are wonderful chopped and mixed into a salad.

Total Time: 20 mins
Servings 4 servings

Ingredients
- 1 tsp Dijon Mustard
- 1 1/2 tbsp red wine vinegar

- 1 tbsp extra virgin olive oil
- 2 tsp fresh chopped parsley
- kosher salt and pepper to taste
- 1 pound thin asparagus, tough ends trimmed off

Instructions

- In a medium bowl, whisk mustard, vinegar and 1 tbsp oil. Add parsley and season with salt and pepper.
- Steam or boil asparagus for 2-3 minutes until cooked and tender. Drain and run under cold water to stop the cooking.
- Transfer asparagus to a serving dish and drizzle with the vinaigrette.
- Can be served warm or chilled.

Nutrition Info

Serving: ¼

Calories: 57kcal

Carbohydrates: 5.5g

Protein: 2.5g

Fat: 3.5g

Polyunsaturated Fat: 0g

Monounsaturated Fat: 0g

Trans Fat: 0g

Sodium: 92.5mg

Potassium: 0mg

Fiber: 2.5g

Sugar: 0.5g

16 Ham and Swiss Omelet

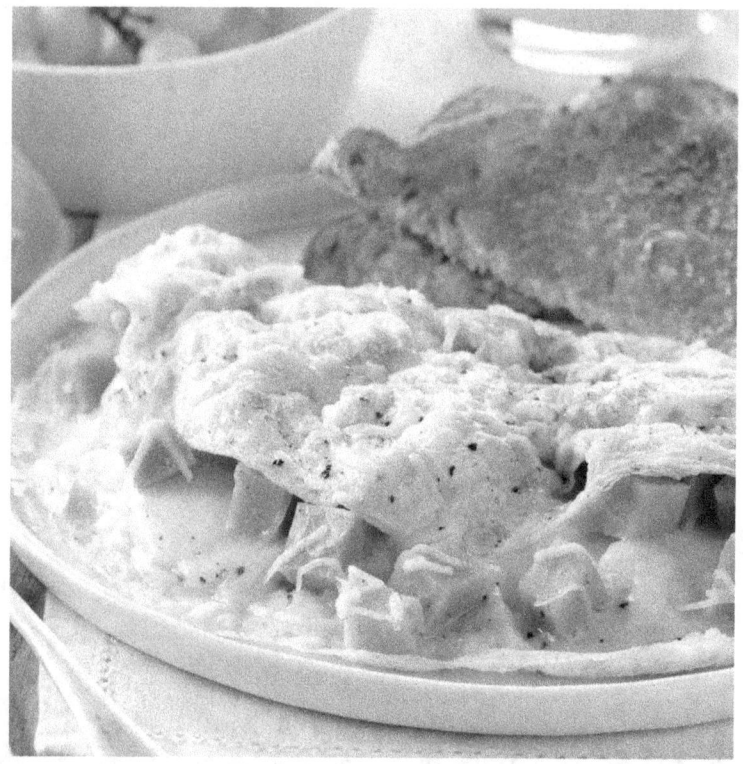

This easy omelet will be a snap to fix for breakfast or dinner.

Prep/Cook Time: 20 min.
1 serving

Ingredients

- 1 tablespoon butter
- 3 eggs
- 3 tablespoons water

- 1/8 teaspoon salt
- 1/8 teaspoon pepper
- 1/2 cup cubed fully cooked ham
- 1/4 cup shredded Swiss cheese

Instructions

- In a small nonstick skillet, melt butter over medium-high heat. Whisk the eggs, water, salt and pepper. Add egg mixture to skillet (mixture should set immediately at edges).
- As eggs set, push cooked edges toward the center, letting uncooked portion flow underneath. When the eggs are set, place ham on one side and sprinkle with cheese; fold other side over filling. Slide omelet onto a plate.

Nutrition Info

1 omelet: 530 calories

40g fat (19g saturated fat)

726mg cholesterol

1551mg sodium

4g carbohydrate (2g sugars, 0 fiber)

39g protein.

17 Feta Asparagus Frittata

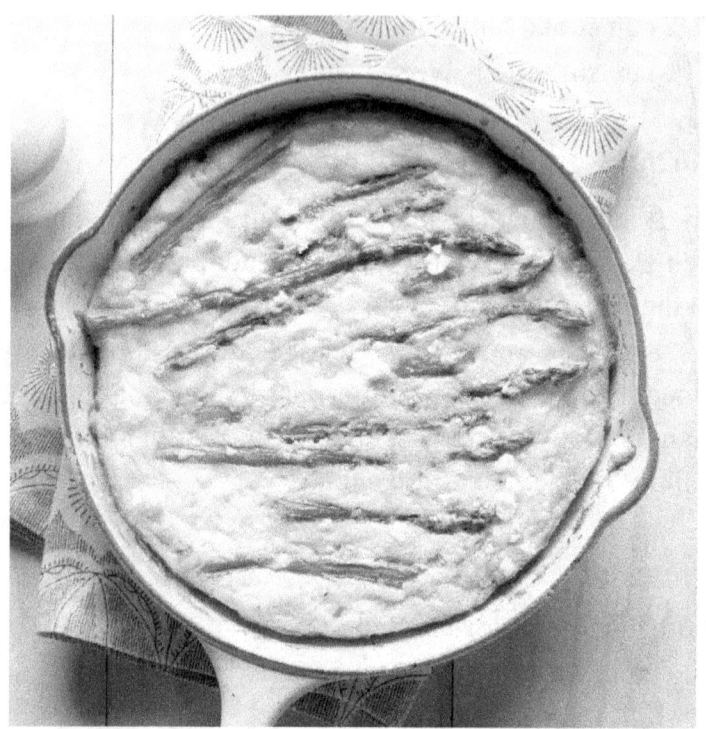

Asparagus and feta cheese come together to make this frittata extra special. Perfect for a lazy Sunday or to serve with a tossed salad for a light lunch.

Prep/Cook Time: 30 min.
2 servings

Ingredients

- 12 fresh asparagus spears, trimmed
- 6 large eggs

- 2 tablespoons heavy whipping cream
- Dash salt
- Dash pepper
- 1 tablespoon olive oil
- 2 green onions, chopped
- 1 garlic clove, minced
- 1/2 cup crumbled feta cheese

Instructions

- Preheat oven to 350°. Place 1/2 in. of water and asparagus in a large skillet; bring to a boil. Cook, covered, until asparagus is crisp-tender, 3-5 minutes; drain. Cool slightly.
- In a bowl, whisk together eggs, cream, salt and pepper. Chop two asparagus spears. In an 8-in. cast-iron or other ovenproof skillet, heat oil over medium heat until hot. Saute green onions, garlic and chopped asparagus 1 minute. Stir in egg mixture; cook, covered, over medium heat until eggs are nearly set, 3-5 minutes. Top with whole asparagus spears and cheese.
- Bake until eggs are completely set, 7-9 minutes.

Nutrition Info

1/2 frittata: 425 calories
31g fat (12g saturated fat)
590mg cholesterol
1231mg sodium
8g carbohydrate (3g sugars, 3g fiber)
27g protein.

18 Denver Omelet Salad

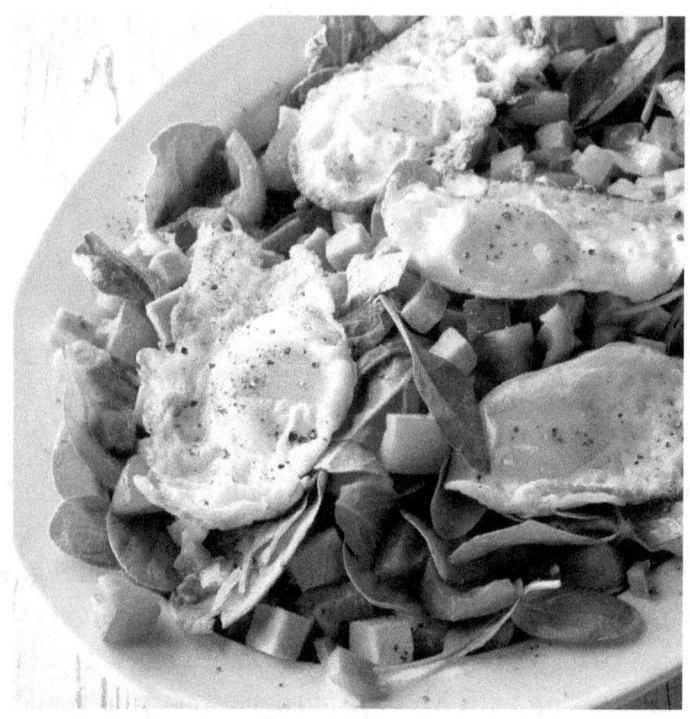

Prep/Cook Time: 25 min.

4 servings

Ingredients

- 8 cups fresh baby spinach
- 1 cup chopped tomatoes
- 2 tablespoons olive oil, divided
- 1-1/2 cups chopped fully cooked ham
- 1 small onion, chopped
- 1 small green pepper, chopped

- 4 large eggs
- Salt and pepper to taste

Instructions

- Arrange spinach and tomatoes on a platter; set aside. In a large skillet, heat 1 tablespoon olive oil over medium-high heat. Add ham, onion and green pepper; saute until ham is heated through and vegetables are tender, 5-7 minutes. Spoon over spinach and tomatoes.
- In same skillet, heat remaining olive oil over medium heat. Break eggs, one at a time, into a small cup, then gently slide into skillet. Immediately reduce heat to low; season with salt and pepper. To prepare sunny-side up eggs, cover pan and cook until whites are completely set and yolks thicken but are not hard. Top salad with fried eggs.

Nutrition Info

1 serving: 229 calories

14g fat (3g saturated fat)

217mg cholesterol

756mg sodium

7g carbohydrate (3g sugars, 2g fiber)

20g protein.

19 Broiled Tilapia with Garlic

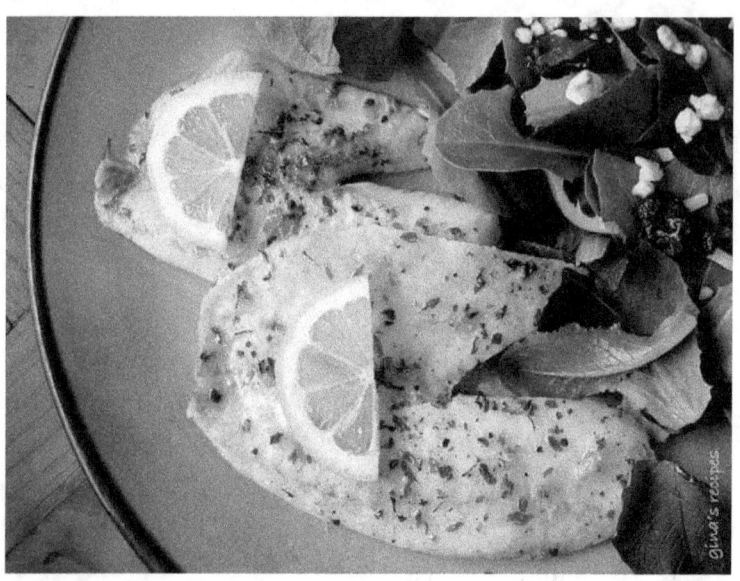

Cook Time: 7 mins

Servings 6 servings

Ingredients

- 6 tilapia fillets, 6oz
- 2 cloves garlic, crushed
- 3 tsp extra virgin olive oil
- 1 tsp oregano
- 1 tsp parsley
- salt and pepper
- 1 lemon

Instructions

- Wash fish and pat dry.
- Line broiler pan with tin foil.
- Place fish on the tin foil and season with salt, pepper, oregano, and parsley.
- Drizzle with olive oil and top with crushed garlic.
- Set broiler to low and place fish about 8 inches from the flame.
- Cook until fish is cooked through, about 7 minutes (be careful not to burn garlic).
- Serve with freshly squeezed lemon juice.

Nutrition Info

Serving: 1filet

Calories: 197.3kcal

Carbohydrates: 2.4g

Protein: 34.6g

Fat: 6.5g

Polyunsaturated Fat: 0g

Monounsaturated Fat: 0g

Trans Fat: 0g

Sodium: 129.5mg

Potassium: 0mg

Fiber: 1g

Sugar: 0g

20 Hard-Boiled Eggs

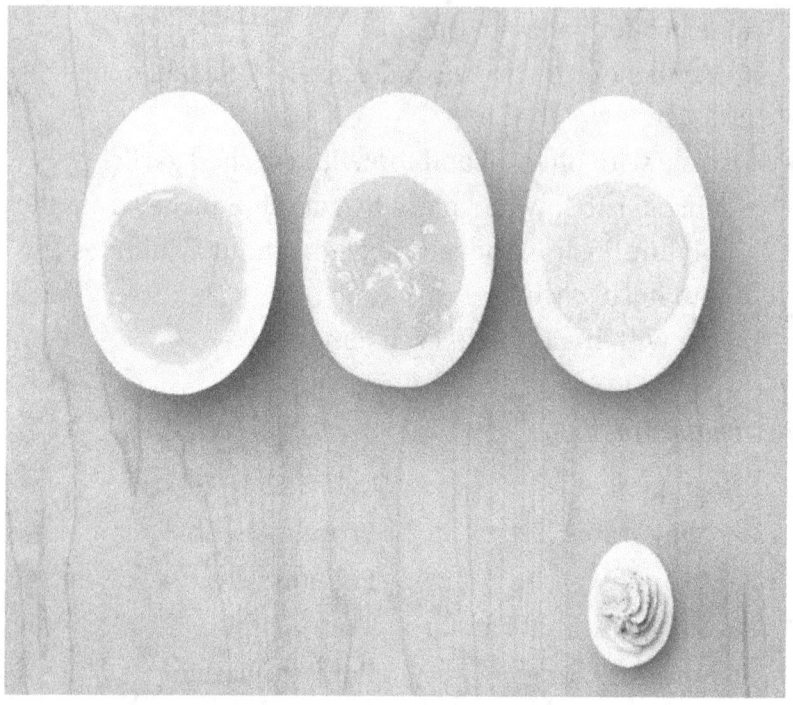

In the kitchen, it's important to start with something simple, like how to cook hard boiled eggs. Use these in plenty of recipes or eat plain for a quick protein fix.

Prep: 20 min. + cooling
12 servings

Ingredients

- 12 large eggs
- Cold water

Instructions

- Place eggs in a single layer in a large saucepan; add enough cold water to cover by 1 in. Cover and quickly bring to a boil. Remove from the heat. Let stand for 15 minutes for large eggs (18 minutes for extra-large eggs and 12 minutes for medium eggs).
- Rinse eggs in cold water and place in ice water until completely cooled. Drain and refrigerate.

Nutrition Info

1 each: 75 calories   5g fat (2g saturated fat)
213mg cholesterol   63mg sodium
1g carbohydrate   6g protein.

21 Cuban Picadillo

This Cuban Picadillo recipe is my family's favorite! It's really quick and easy to make, I make it a few times a month and make enough so we have leftovers!

Total Time: 30 mins
Servings 6 Servings

Ingredients

- 1/2 large chopped onion
- 2 cloves garlic, minced
- 1 to mato, chopped
- 1/2 pepper, finely chopped
- 2 tbsp cilantro

- 1-1/2 lb 93% lean ground beef
- 4 oz 1/2 can tomato sauce (I like Goya, check label for Keto)
- kosher salt
- fresh ground pepper
- 1 tsp ground cumin
- 1-2 bay leaf
- 2 tbsp alcaparrado, capers or green olives would work too

Instructions

- Brown meat on high heat in large sauté pan and season with salt and pepper. Use a wooden spoon to break the meat up into small pieces. When meat is no longer pink, drain all juice from pan.
- Meanwhile, while meat is cooking, chop onion, garlic, pepper, tomato and cilantro.
- Add to the meat and continue cooking on a low flame. Add alcaparrado and about 2 tbsp of the brine (the juice from the olives, this adds great flavor) cumin, bay leaf, and more salt if needed. Add tomato sauce and 1/4 cup of water and mix well. Reduce heat and simmer covered about 20 minutes.

Nutrition Info

Serving: 1/2 cup   Calories: 207kcal
Carbohydrates: 5g   Protein: 25g
Fat: 8.5

22 Eggs with Scallions and Tomatoes

Servings 2 servings

Ingredients

- 2 large eggs
- 3 large egg whites
- 4 diced scallions
- 1 large diced tomato
- 1 tsp olive oil
- salt and pepper

Instructions

- Heat olive oil in a frying pan on a medium-low flame and add scallions and tomatoes.
- Mix eggs in a bowl and season with salt and pepper.
- Add the eggs to the frying pan and stir as they cook 2-3 minutes.

Nutrition Info

Serving: ½	Calories: 155kcal
Carbohydrates: 8.5g	Protein: 13.9g
Fat: 7.7g	Polyunsaturated Fat: 0g
Monounsaturated Fat: 0g	Trans Fat: 0g
Potassium: 0mg	Fiber: 2.3g

23 Pan Seared Shrimp

4 servings

Ingredients

- 2 tsp vegetable oil
- 1 1/2 lbs shrimp, peeled and deveined (weight after peeled)
- 1/4 tsp salt
- 1/4 tsp ground black pepper
- 1/4 tsp crushed red pepper
- 2 tbsp dry parsley
- lemon wedges

Instructions

- Heat 1 tsp oil in 12 inch skillet over high heat until smoking.
- Meanwhile, toss shrimp with salt, pepper, parsley and crushed red pepper.
- Add half of the shrimp to the pan in single layer and cook until edges turn pink, about 1 minute.
- Remove pan from heat, flip shrimp using tongs and let it stand about 30 seconds until all of the shrimp is opaque except for the center.
- Transfer to a plate and repeat with the second batch and the remaining teaspoon of oil.
- After second batch has stood off the heat, add the first batch to the pan and toss to combine.
- Cover skillet and let shrimp stand for 1 - 2 minutes.
- Shrimp will now be cooked through.
- Serve immediately with lemon wedges.

Nutrition Info

Serving: ¼

Calories: 148.6kcal

Carbohydrates: 0.5g

Protein: 26.8g

Fat: 3.7g

Polyunsaturated Fat: 0g

Monounsaturated Fat: 0g

Trans Fat: 0g

Potassium: 0mg

Fiber: 0.3g

24 Tomato and Green Pepper Omelet

Fresh green pepper, onion and tomato give this savory omelet garden-fresh flavors. You can easily vary it based on the fresh ingredients you have on hand.

Prep/Cook Time: 20 min

1 serving

Ingredients

- 1/3 cup chopped green pepper
- 2 tablespoons chopped onion
- 2 teaspoons olive oil
- 1 tablespoon butter
- 3 eggs
- 3 tablespoons water
- 1/8 teaspoon salt
- 1/8 teaspoon pepper
- 1/3 cup chopped tomato

Instructions

- In a small nonstick skillet, saute green pepper and onion in oil until tender. Remove from skillet and set aside.
- In the same skillet, melt butter over medium-high heat. Whisk the eggs, water, salt and pepper. Add egg mixture to skillet (mixture should set immediately at edges).
- As eggs set, push cooked edges toward the center, letting uncooked portion flow underneath. When the eggs are set, spoon green pepper mixture and tomato on one side; fold other side over filling. Slide omelet onto a plate.

Nutrition Info

1 omelet: 424 calories
665mg cholesterol
20g protein

35g fat (13g saturated fat)
591mg sodium
8g carbohydrate

25 Greek Veggie Omelet

Prep/Cook Time: 20 min.
2 servings

Ingredients

- 4 large eggs
- 2 tablespoons fat-free milk
- 1/8 teaspoon salt
- 3 teaspoons olive oil, divided
- 2 cups sliced baby portobello mushrooms
- 1/4 cup finely chopped onion

- 1 cup fresh baby spinach
- 3 tablespoons crumbled feta cheese
- 2 tablespoons sliced ripe olives
- Freshly ground pepper

Instructions

- Whisk together eggs, milk and salt. In a large nonstick skillet, heat 2 teaspoons oil over medium-high heat; saute mushrooms and onion until golden brown, 5-6 minutes. Stir in spinach until wilted; remove from pan.
- In same pan, heat remaining oil over medium-low heat. Pour in egg mixture. As eggs set, push cooked portions toward the center, letting uncooked eggs flow underneath. When eggs are thickened and no liquid egg remains, spoon vegetables on one side; sprinkle with cheese and olives. Fold to close; cut in half to serve. Sprinkle with pepper.

Nutrition Info

1/2 omelet: 271 calories

378mg cholesterol

7g carbohydrate

19g fat (5g saturated fat)

475mg sodium

18g protein

26 Herb & Cheese Scrambled Eggs

Prep/Cook Time: 15 min.
4 servings

Ingredients

- 8 large eggs
- 1/2 cup 2% milk or half-and-half cream
- 4 ounces cream cheese, softened
- 1 tablespoon minced fresh parsley
- 1 tablespoon minced chives
- 1/2 teaspoon minced fresh thyme
- 1/8 to 1/4 teaspoon salt
- 1/8 teaspoon white pepper
- 1 tablespoon butter
- Additional minced fresh herbs

Instructions

- Whisk together the first eight ingredients. In a large nonstick skillet, heat butter over medium heat.
- Pour in egg mixture; cook and stir until eggs are thickened and no liquid egg remains. Sprinkle with additional minced herbs.

Nutrition Info

1 serving: 284 calories
411mg cholesterol
4g carbohydrate

23g fat (11g saturated fat)
343mg sodium
15g protein.

27 Shiitake and Manchego Scramble

This savory breakfast dish takes everyday scrambled eggs up a few notches. The rich flavor is so satisfying in the morning, and it's even better served with buttery toasted Italian bread.

Prep/Total Time: 25 min.
8 servings

Ingredients

- 2 tablespoons extra virgin olive oil, divided
- 1/2 cup diced onion
- 1/2 cup diced sweet red pepper
- 2 cups thinly sliced fresh shiitake mushrooms (about 4 ounces)
- 1 teaspoon prepared horseradish
- 8 large eggs, beaten
- 1 cup heavy whipping cream
- 1 cup shredded Manchego cheese
- 1 teaspoon kosher salt
- 1 teaspoon coarsely ground pepper

Instructions

- In a large nonstick skillet, heat 1 tablespoon olive oil over medium heat. Add onion and red pepper; cook and stir until crisp-tender, 2-3 minutes. Add mushrooms; cook and stir until tender, 3-4 minutes. Stir in horseradish; cook 2 minutes more.

- In a small bowl, whisk together remaining ingredients and remaining olive oil. Pour into skillet; cook and stir until eggs are thickened and no liquid egg remains.

Nutrition Info

1 serving: 274 calories

24g fat (12g saturated fat)

234mg cholesterol

405mg sodium

4g carbohydrate

11g protein.

28 Skinny Low-Yolk Egg Salad

What to do with all your leftover Easter eggs? Make this easy guiltless egg salad made with mostly egg whites and scallions. Serve this on your favorite whole grain bread or enjoy on lettuce cups.

Prep Time: 15 mins

Total Time: 15 mins

Servings 2 servings

Ingredients

- 4 hard boiled eggs, peeled
- 4 tsp Hellman's light mayonnaise
- 1/2 tsp dijon mustard
- 2 tbsp chopped green scallions or chives
- salt and fresh pepper to taste

Instructions

- Separate the yolks from the egg whites and discard 3 of the yolks.

- Chop eggs and combine with mayonnaise, dijon mustard, scallions, salt and pepper.

Nutrition Info

Serving: 1/2 of salad

Calories: 81kcal

Carbohydrates: 1g

Protein: 9.5g

Fat: 4.5g

Saturated Fat: 2g

Polyunsaturated Fat: 0g

Monounsaturated Fat: 0g

Trans Fat: 0g

29 Carne Bistec - Colombian Steak with Onions and Tomatoes

Servings 6 servings

Ingredients

- 1-1/2 lbs grass fed sirloin tip steak, sliced very thin
- salt to taste
- garlic powder to taste
- cumin to taste
- 4 tsp olive oil
- 1 medium onion, sliced thin or chopped
- 1 very large tomato or 2 medium tomatoes, sliced thin or chopped

Instructions

- Season steak with salt and garlic powder.
- Heat a large frying pan until VERY HOT.

- Add 2 tsp of oil then half of the steak and cook less than a minute on each side.
- Set steak aside, add another teaspoon of oil and cook remaining steak.
- Set aside.
- Reduce heat to medium, add another teaspoon of oil and add the onions.
- Cook 2 minutes, then add the tomatoes.
- Season with salt, pepper and cumin and reduce heat to medium-low.
- Add about 1/4 cup of water and simmer a few minutes to create a sauce, add more water if needed and taste adjust seasoning as needed.
- Return the steak to the pan along with the drippings, combine well and remove from heat.
- Serve over rice or for a low carb option with a sunny-side up egg on top.

Nutrition Info

Serving: 3 oz steak + onions tomatoes
Calories: 182.9kcal
Carbohydrates: 3g
Protein: 25.2g, Fat: 7.2g
Polyunsaturated Fat: 0g
Monounsaturated Fat: 0g
Trans Fat: 0g
Potassium: 0mg
Fiber: 0.7g

30 Sauteed Collard Greens with Bacon

Collard greens sliced thin sauteed with bacon, garlic and oil. A perfect side dish for Brazilian black beans or black eyed peas with ham.

Prep Time: 5 mins
Cook Time: 15 mins
Total Time: 20 mins
Servings 4 servings

Ingredients

- 1 tbsp olive oil
- 1 slice bacon, chopped
- 3 cloves garlic, chopped
- 1 bunch collard greens, washed and dried
- salt

Instructions

- Remove the tough stems that run down the center of the leaf.
- Stack a few leaves, roll and slice into thin strips.
- In a large saute pan, heat bacon on low heat.
- When bacon fat melts, add oil and garlic, saute until golden, about a minute.
- Add chopped collards to the pan, season with salt and cover.
- Simmer covered until tender, about 10 minutes, stirring occasionally.

Nutrition Info

Serving: 1/4th   Calories: 72.9kcal

Carbohydrates: 6.8g   Protein: 3.1g

Fat: 4.5g   Saturated Fat: 0.8g

Polyunsaturated Fat: 0g   Monounsaturated Fat: 0g

Trans Fat: 0g   Cholesterol: 1.3mg

Sodium: 68mg   Potassium: 0mg

Fiber: 2.4g   Sugar: 0.5g

31 Steamed Asparagus with Poached Eggs

Poached eggs, asparagus, kosher salt, fresh pepper and shaved Pecorino Romano. This simple egg dish is delicious for breakfast, lunch or brunch. You can serve this with whole grain toast on the side.

Total Time: 45 mins
Servings 4 servings

Ingredients

- 2 bunches medium sized asparagus, tough ends removed (about 36 medium spears)
- 4 large eggs
- kosher salt and fresh pepper
- 2 tbsp Parmigiano Reggiano, freshly shaved

Instructions

- Steam asparagus until tender-crisp, then run under cool water for a few seconds to stop the cooking.
- Drain and divide asparagus between four plates.
- Poach eggs in an egg poacher or following these steps for poaching eggs without one.
- Remove with a slotted spoon and place each egg on top of each plate of asparagus.
- Top with freshly grated salt, pepper and Parmigiano Reggiano. Enjoy!!

Nutrition Info

Serving: 1egg with asparagus

Calories: 114kcal

Carbohydrates: 7g

Protein: 10.5g

Fat: 6g

Polyunsaturated Fat: 0g

Monounsaturated Fat: 0g

Trans Fat: 0g

Potassium: 0mg

Fiber: 3g

32 Shrimp Salad on Cucumber Slices

Prp/Cook Time: 30 minutes
Servings 30 servings

Ingredients

- 3/4 lb cooked shrimp, peeled (weight after peeled)
- 2 celery stalks, chopped
- 1 tbsp red onion, chopped
- 2 tbsp light mayonnaise, I used Hellmann's, check label for Keto
- 1 tbsp fat free Greek yogurt, full fat for Keto
- Seasoning salt or adobo seasoning
- salt and fresh ground pepper
- 30 thin slices cucumber, about 1 large
- chopped chives for garnish

Instructions

- Combine shrimp, celery, onion, mayonnaise, yogurt, and season to taste with seasoning salt or adobo and pepper.
- Arrange cucumbers on a platter, season with salt and top each slice with a heaping tablespoon of shrimp salad.
- Top with chopped chives for garnish.

Nutrition Info

Servings: 4
1/4 cucumber
3 pts Calories: 117.5
Protein: 18.8 g
Fiber: 1.0 g

Serving Size: 1/4 lb salad
Old Points: 2 pts
Fat: 2.8 g
Carb: 3.7 g

33 Skinny Tzatziki

Prep Time: 15 mins
Total Time: 1 hr 15 mins
Servings 8

Ingredients

- 8 oz fat-free Greek yogurt, I used Fage, use full fat for Keto
- 1 small cucumber, peeled and seeded (1 cup grated and squeezed dry)
- 1 clove garlic, crushed
- 1 tsp lemon juice
- 1 tbsp fresh dill, chopped
- 1 tbsp fresh chives, chopped
- kosher salt and fresh pepper

Instructions

- Strain the yogurt using a metal strainer or a coffee filter for a few hours to remove as much liquid as possible. Set aside.
- Scoop seeds out of the cucumber with a small spoon. Place cucumber in a mini food processor or grate with a box cheese grater. Drain the liquid from the cucumber in a metal strainer and sprinkle with a little salt (this helps release the liquid). You may want to use the back of a spoon to help squeeze out any excess liquid.
- Combine strained cucumber, garlic, yogurt, salt, pepper, lemon juice, dill, chives and refrigerate at least 1 hour before serving.
- Makes about 2 cups. Store in refrigerator for about a week.

Nutrition Info

Serving: 1/4 cup

Calories: 18kcal

Carbohydrates: 1.7g

Protein: 2.6g

Fat: 0g

Polyunsaturated Fat: 0g

Monounsaturated Fat: 0g

Trans Fat: 0g

Potassium: 0mg

Fiber: 0.1g

34 Spaghetti Squash Pesto with Tomatoes

Prep Time: 10 mins

Cook Time: 10 mins

Total Time: 20 mins

Servings 4 servings

Ingredients

- 1 small spaghetti squash
- 15 large basil leaves
- 1 small clove garlic
- 1/4 cup olive oil
- 3 tbsp Parmigiano-Reggiano
- salt and fresh pepper
- 1 to mato, diced

Instructions

- Cut squash in half lengthwise, scoop out seeds and fibers.
- Place in a microwave safe dish and cover.
- Microwave 8-9 minutes.

- Remove from the microwave and scoop out flesh with a fork into a large bowl.
- In a small blender combine basil, garlic, olive oil, parmesan cheese, salt a pepper and puree until smooth.
- Combine pesto with two cups spaghetti squash (save any remaining squash for another recipe).
- Add tomatoes and season with additional salt and pepper.

Nutrition Info

Serving: 1/4th	Calories: 165.4kcal
Carbohydrates: 6.9g	Protein: 2.4g
Fat: 14.9g	Saturated Fat: 2.6g
Polyunsaturated Fat: 0g	Monounsaturated Fat: 0g
Trans Fat: 0g	Cholesterol: 3mg
Sodium: 86.7mg	Potassium: 0mg
Fiber: 1.5g	Sugar: 2g

35 Creamy Parmesan Spinach Dip

Prp/Cook Time: 40 minutes   Servings 8 servings

Ingredients

- 10 oz frozen chopped spinach, thawed and excess liquid squeezed out
- 1/2 cup light sour cream, full fat for Keto
- 5 tbsp light mayonnaise, full fat, check labels for Keto
- 1/3 cup Parmigiano Reggiano
- 1/4 cup scallion, chopped
- fresh pepper to taste

Instructions

- Combine all the ingredients in a medium bowl.
- Can be made one day in advance and stored in the refrigerator.
- Remove from refrigerator 30 minutes before serving.

Nutrition Info

Serving: 1/4 cup   Calories: 79.4kcal

Carbohydrates: 3.3g   Protein: 3.2g

Fat: 6.2g   Polyunsaturated Fat: 0g

Monounsaturated Fat: 0g   Trans Fat: 0g

Potassium: 0mg   Fiber: 0.9g

36 Roasted Broccoli Rabe with Garlic

Broccoli Rabe roasted with chunks of garlic and oil and a touch of crushed red pepper flakes.

Prep Time: 5 mins

Cook Time: 25 mins

Total Time: 30 mins

Servings 4 servings

Ingredients

- 1 large bunch broccoli rabe, rapini, tough stems removed
- 4-5 cloves garlic, smashed
- 2 tbsp olive oil
- salt and fresh pepper
- pinch crushed red pepper flakes, optional

Instructions

- Heat oven to 400°.
- Bring a large pot of salted water to a boil.
- When water boils, add broccoli rabe and blanch one minute.
- Remove from water and DRAIN WELL in a colander.
- Add to a baking dish and mix with garlic, oil, salt, pepper, crushed red pepper flakes.
- Roast 15-20 minutes.

Nutrition Info

Serving: 1/4th

Calories: 72.4kcal

Carbohydrates: 1.7g

Protein: 1.2g

Fat: 7g

Saturated Fat: 1g

Polyunsaturated Fat: 0g

Monounsaturated Fat: 0g

Trans Fat: 0g

Cholesterol: 0mg

Sodium: 14.5mg

Potassium: 0mg

Fiber: 0.8g

Sugar: 0.3g

37 Broiled or Grilled Pollo Sabroso

Prep Time: 15 mins

Total Time: 45 mins

Servings 6 servings

Ingredients

- 6 medium chicken thighs, with bone and skin
- 1 tbsp vinegar
- 2 teaspoons soy sauce, coconut aminos for whole30

- 1 packet Sazon, in Spanish aisle, I prefer Badia brand with no MSG
- 1 teaspoon Adobo, in Spanish aisle
- 1/2 teaspoon garlic powder
- 1/2 teaspoon dried oregano

Instructions

- Season chicken with vinegar and soy sauce.
- Add sazon, 1 teaspoon of adobo, garlic powder, oregano and adobo and mix well. (Don't use your hands or they will turn orange)
- Let chicken marinate at least 15 minutes.
- Broil or grill on low until chicken is cooked through, turning halfway, careful not to burn, about 30 minutes. Enjoy with rice and salad.

Nutrition Info

Serving: 1thigh

Calories: 181kcal

Carbohydrates: 0.5g

Protein: 29.5g

Fat: 6g

Saturated Fat: 1.5g

Polyunsaturated Fat: 0g

Monounsaturated Fat: 0g

Trans Fat: 0g

Cholesterol: 140mg

Sodium: 383.5mg

Potassium: 0mg

Fiber: 0g

Sugar: 0g

38 Cilantro Chicken Salad

This easy chicken salad recipe is made with scallions, cilantro with a hint of lime. It's a tasty twist on traditional chicken salad with some Latin flavor!

Prep Time: 10 mins
Total Time: 15 mins
Servings 2 servings

Ingredients

- 7 oz cooked chicken breast, shredded or diced
- 2 tbsp light mayonnaise, full fat for Keto
- 1 small scallion, chopped
- 2 tsp lime juice
- 2 tbsp chopped cilantro
- kosher salt and pepper
- 1/8 teaspoon garlic powder
- 1/8 teaspoon cumin
- 1/8 teaspoon chile powder
- low sodium chicken broth, check labels for Keto or use bullion

Instructions

- Combine chicken, mayonnaise, scallions, lime juice, and cilantro.
- Season to taste with salt, pepper, garlic powder, cumin, and chile powder.
- Add a little chicken broth if chicken seams too dry, 1 tbsp at a time.

To Poach:

- Cover chicken breast in broth in a small pot, add water if it doesn't cover the chicken.
- Add salt and pepper, a piece of celery and it's leaves (you could add herbs like parsley, garlic, onion, or whatever you want) and bring to a boil. Reduce to a simmer and cook 5 minutes.
- Remove from heat, cover tight and let it sit for 15-20 minutes or until thickest part of the breast registers 160 degrees.
- Chicken will be cooked through. Let it cool and cut into small cubes.

Nutrition Info

Serving: ½	Calories: 163.5kcal
Carbohydrates: 2.5g	Protein: 23g
Fat: 6g	Polyunsaturated Fat: 0g
Monounsaturated Fat: 0g	Trans Fat: 0g
Potassium: 0mg	Fiber: 0.5g

39 Pork Chops with Mushrooms and Shallots

Prep/Cook Time: 50 minutes
Servings 4 servings

Ingredients

- 1 tsp butter or ghee
- 4 pork loin chops, bone-in, trimmed or 1 lb (boneless)
- 1/2 tsp kosher salt
- fresh black pepper

- 1/4 cup chopped shallots
- 1 cup low sodium chicken stock
- 10 oz sliced baby bella mushrooms
- 1 tbsp Dijon mustard
- 2 tbsp chopped, fresh parsley

Instructions

- In a large frying pan heat the butter over moderately low heat.
- Season pork with salt and pepper.
- Raise heat to medium and add the chops to the pan and sauté for 7 minutes.
- Turn and cook until chops are browned and done to medium, about 7-8 minutes longer or until the pork reads 160F in the center.
- Remove the chops and put in a warm spot.
- Add shallots to the pan and cook, stirring, until soft, about 3 minutes.
- Add the stock to deglaze the pan, stir in the mustard, 1 tbsp parsley, then add mushrooms, season with fresh pepper and cook about 3 minutes, or until mushrooms are done.
- Put the chops on a platter and pour the mushroom sauce over the meat, top with remaining parsley.

Nutrition Info

Serving: 1chop
Carbohydrates: 4.3g
Fat: 9.5g
Monounsaturated Fat: 0g
Potassium: 0mg

Calories: 180kcal
Protein: 18.5g
Polyunsaturated Fat: 0g
Trans Fat: 0g
Fiber: 0.9g

40 Grilled Chicken with Spinach and Melted Mozzarella

Grilled chicken topped with sauteed garlicky spinach, mozzarella and roasted peppers – a quick and easy chicken dish your family will love!

Servings 6 Servings

Ingredients

- 24 oz 3 large chicken breasts sliced in half lengthwise to make 6
- kosher salt and pepper to taste
- 1 tsp olive oil
- 3 cloves garlic, crushed
- 10 oz frozen spinach, drained
- 3 oz shredded part skim mozzarella
- 1/2 cup roasted red pepper, sliced in strips (packed in water)
- olive oil spray

Instructions

- Preheat oven to 400°F. Season chicken with salt and pepper. Lightly spray a grill or grill pan with oil. Cook chicken until no longer pink, about 2 to 3 minutes per side.
- Heat a skillet over medium heat. Add oil and garlic, sauté a 30 seconds, add spinach, salt and pepper. Cook until heated through, 2 to 3 minutes.
- Place chicken on a baking sheet , divide spinach evenly between the 6 pieces and place on top. Top each with 1/2 oz mozzarella, roasted peppers and bake until melted, about 3 minutes.

Nutrition Info

Serving: 1piece

Calories: 195kcal

Carbohydrates: 3.5g

Protein: 31g

Fat: 6g, Saturated Fat: 2g

Polyunsaturated Fat: 0g

Monounsaturated Fat: 0g

Trans Fat: 0g

Cholesterol: 91mg

Sodium: 183mg

Potassium: 0mg

Fiber: 1.5g

Sugar: 0.5g

41 Pepper and Fresh Herb Frittata

Peppers add "zing" to this wonderful egg dish, chock-full of herby seasoning. It's simple to put together for breakfast or brunch.

Prep/Total Time: 30 min.

6 servings

Ingredients

- 12 large eggs
- 2 tablespoons minced fresh chives
- 2 tablespoons minced fresh parsley
- 2 teaspoons minced fresh basil or 1/2 teaspoon dried basil
- 2 teaspoons minced fresh oregano or 1/2 teaspoon dried oregano
- 1 teaspoon salt
- 1/4 teaspoon pepper
- 3 tablespoons olive oil
- 1/2 cup sliced pickled peppers
- 1/2 cup crumbled goat cheese

Instructions

- Preheat broiler. In a large bowl, whisk eggs, herbs, salt and pepper until blended.
- In a 10-in. broiler-safe skillet, heat oil over medium-low heat. Pour in egg mixture. Cook, covered, 10-12 minutes or until nearly set. Top with pickled peppers and cheese.
- Broil 4-5 in. from heat 3-4 minutes or until eggs are completely set. Let stand 5 minutes. Cut into wedges.

Nutrition Info

1 wedge: 234 calories

19g fat (6g saturated fat)

384mg cholesterol

708mg sodium

2g carbohydrate

14g protein.

42 Eggs with Scallions and Tomatoes

Servings 2 servings

Ingredients

- 2 large eggs
- 3 large egg whites
- 4 diced scallions
- 1 large diced tomato
- 1 tsp olive oil
- salt and pepper

Instructions

- Heat olive oil in a frying pan on a medium-low flame and add scallions and tomatoes.
- Mix eggs in a bowl and season with salt and pepper.
- Add the eggs to the frying pan and stir as they cook 2-3 minutes.

Nutrition Info

Serving: ½	Calories: 155kcal
Carbohydrates: 8.5g	Protein: 13.9g
Fat: 7.7g	Polyunsaturated Fat: 0g
Monounsaturated Fat: 0g	Trans Fat: 0g
Potassium: 0mg	Fiber: 2.3g

43 Greek Breakfast Casserole

This is a great dish for a Sunday brunch, or you can cut it into six pieces and freeze it to have as a quick and easy breakfast any day of the week. I also like to make it with broccoli, carrots, green onions, Canadian bacon and sharp cheddar cheese; the variations are nearly endless!

Prep: 35 min. Bake: 45 min. + standing
6 servings

Ingredients

- 1/2 pound Italian turkey sausage links, casings removed
- 1/2 cup chopped green pepper
- 1 shallot, chopped

- 1 cup water-packed artichoke hearts, rinsed, drained and chopped
- 1 cup chopped fresh broccoli
- 1/3 cup sun-dried tomatoes (not packed in oil), chopped
- 6 large eggs
- 6 large egg whites
- 3 tablespoons fat-free milk
- 1/2 teaspoon Italian seasoning
- 1/4 teaspoon garlic powder
- 1/4 teaspoon pepper
- 1/3 cup crumbled feta cheese

Instructions

- Preheat oven to 350°. In a large skillet, cook sausage, green pepper and shallot over medium heat until sausage is no longer pink, breaking up sausage into crumbles, 8-10 minutes; drain. Transfer mixture to an 8-in. square baking dish coated with cooking spray. Top with artichokes, broccoli and sun-dried tomatoes.
- In a large bowl, whisk eggs, egg whites, milk and seasonings until blended; pour over top. Sprinkle with feta.
- Bake, uncovered, until a knife inserted in the center comes out clean, 45-50 minutes. Let stand 10 minutes before serving.
- Freeze option: Cool baked casserole; cover and freeze. To use, partially thaw in refrigerator overnight. Remove from refrigerator 30 minutes before baking. Preheat oven to 325°. Bake casserole as directed until heated through and a thermometer inserted in center reads 165°.

Nutrition Info

1 piece: 179 calories
229mg cholesterol
8g carbohydrate

9g fat (3g saturated fat)
435mg sodium
17g protein.

44 Basil Green Goddess Dressing Recipe

Servings 16 servings

Ingredients

- 1/2 cup light mayonnaise, such as Hellman's (regular for Keto)
- 1/2 cup scallions, chopped
- 1/2 cup chopped fresh basil, packed
- 1/8 cup fresh squeezed lemon juice, 1 lemon
- 1 clove garlic, chopped
- 1 tsp kosher salt
- 1/2 tsp freshly ground black pepper
- 1 tsp anchovy paste
- 1/2 cup light sour cream, full fat for Keto

Instructions

- Place all ingredients except for sour cream in a blender and blend until smooth.
- Add sour cream and process until blended.
- Keep refrigerated until serving.

Nutrition Info

Serving: 2tbsp

Calories: 60.3kcal

Carbohydrates: 2.9g

Protein: 1.3g

Fat: 4.9g

Polyunsaturated Fat: 0g

Monounsaturated Fat: 0g

Trans Fat: 0g

Potassium: 0mg

Fiber: 0.3g

45 Creamy Shrimp and Celery Salad

4 servings

Ingredients

- 16 oz large cooked shrimp, peeled
- 2 medium cucumbers, peeled and sliced
- 1 large celery stalk, sliced thin
- 1/4 cup low fat sour cream, regular for Keto
- 2 tbsp lite mayonnaise, regular for Keto
- 2 tbsp lime juice
- 1 tsp Old Bay seasoning
- salt to taste

Instructions

- In a medium bowl, combine sour cream, mayonnaise, lime juice, Old Bay and salt.
- Add shrimp, celery, cucumbers and mix.
- Refrigerate until ready to serve.

Nutrition Info

Calories: 160.2kcal   Carbohydrates: 3.8g

Protein: 25.1g   Fat: 4.5g

46 Broiled Salmon with Rosemary

Juicy salmon with rosemary, lemon and garlic, takes minutes to prepare which is always perfect for busy weeknights.

Total Time: 30 mins

Servings 4 servings

Ingredients

- 24 oz or 4 pieces of salmon
- olive oil spray
- 2 tsp fresh lemon juice
- 2 tsp fresh, chopped rosemary
- 2 cloves garlic, minced
- salt and fresh pepper to taste

Instructions

- Combine lemon juice, rosemary, salt, pepper and garlic. Brush mixture onto fish.
- Spray the rack of a broiler pan with olive oil spray and arrange the fish on it.
- Broil 4" from the heat until fish flakes easily when tested with a fork, approx. 4-6 minutes per 1/2" of thickness.

- If fish is more than 1" thick, gently turn it halfway through broiling.

Nutrition Info

Serving: 1piece salmon

Calories: 245kcal

Carbohydrates: 1g

Protein: 34g

Fat: 11g, Saturated Fat: 1.5g

Polyunsaturated Fat: 0g

Monounsaturated Fat: 0g

Trans Fat: 0g

Cholesterol: 94mg

Sodium: 74.5mg

Potassium: 0mg

Fiber: 0.1g

Sugar: 0.1g

47 Filipino BBQ Pork Skewers

If you want to make a delicious recipe at your next BBQ that will wow everyone, these Filipino BBQ Skewers are it. I've tried this marinade on beef, pork and chicken and it's great on everything!

Prep Time: 15 mins
Cook Time: 10 mins
Total Time: 25 mins

Ingredients

- 2.5 lb pork country style ribs
- All fat trimmed
- Cut into 1" x 1" cubes

For the marinade:

- 6 oz 7-up
- 1/2 cup soy sauce
- 1/2 cup white vinegar
- 1 lemon, juice of
- 1/3 cup brown sugar
- 6 cloves garlic, crushed
- 1 tsp black pepper
- crushed red pepper flakes, optional

Instructions

- Mix all ingredients in a large non-reactive bowl and marinate the meat overnight.
- If using wooden skewers, soak in water at least an hour so they don't burn on the grill.
- Thread the meat onto skewers and grill.
- Discard unused marinade.
- Enjoy!

Nutrition Info

Serving: 4oz

Calories: 135kcal

Carbohydrates: 7g

Protein: 14.5g

Fat: 6g, Saturated Fat: 2g

Polyunsaturated Fat: 0g

Monounsaturated Fat: 0g

Trans Fat: 0g

Cholesterol: 45mg

Sodium: 499mg

Potassium: 0mg

48 Cheesy Chive Omelet

Fuel up for the day with eggs for breakfast. When you want a change, try the other omelet ideas at the end of the recipe.

Prep/Cook Time: 15 min.
2 servings

Ingredients

- 3 large eggs
- 2 tablespoons water
- 1/8 teaspoon salt
- Dash pepper
- 1 tablespoon minced fresh chives
- 1 tablespoon butter
- 1/4 to 1/2 cup shredded cheddar cheese

Instructions

- In a small bowl, whisk eggs, water, salt and pepper. Stir in chives.
- In a small nonstick skillet, heat butter over medium-high heat. Pour in egg mixture. Mixture should set immediately at edges. As eggs set, push cooked portions toward the center, letting uncooked eggs flow underneath.
- When eggs are thickened and no liquid egg remains, sprinkle cheese on one side; fold omelet in half. Cut omelet in half; slide onto plates.

Nutrition Info

1/2 omelet: 216 calories
309mg cholesterol
1g carbohydrate

18g fat (9g saturated fat)
392mg sodium
13g protein.

49 Avocado Scrambled Eggs

Bacon and avocado blend nicely in these special eggs. They're easy perfection for breakfast

Prep/Cook Time: 10 min.
6 servings

Ingredients

- 8 large eggs
- 1/2 cup whole milk
- 1/2 teaspoon salt
- 1/4 teaspoon pepper
- 1 medium ripe avocado, peeled and cubed
- 2 tablespoons butter
- 6 bacon strips, cooked and crumbled

Instructions

- In a bowl, beat eggs. Add milk, salt and pepper; stir in avocado. In a skillet over medium heat, melt butter. Add egg mixture; cook and stir gently until the eggs are completely set. Sprinkle with bacon.

Nutrition Info

1 each: 233 calories

302mg cholesterol

4g carbohydrate

19g fat (7g saturated fat)

434mg sodium

12g protein.

50 Calico Scrambled Eggs

Prep/Cook Time: 15 min.

4 servings

Ingredients

- 8 large eggs
- 1/4 cup 2% milk
- 1/8 to 1/4 teaspoon dill weed
- 1/8 to 1/4 teaspoon salt
- 1/8 to 1/4 teaspoon pepper
- 1 tablespoon butter
- 1/2 cup chopped green pepper
- 1/4 cup chopped onion
- 1/2 cup chopped fresh tomato

Instructions

- In a bowl, whisk the first five ingredients until blended. In a 12-in. nonstick skillet, heat butter over medium-high heat. Add green pepper and onion; cook and stir until tender. Remove from pan.
- In same pan, pour in egg mixture; cook and stir over medium heat until eggs begin to thicken. Add tomato and pepper

mixture; cook until heated through and no liquid egg remains, stirring gently.

Nutrition Info

1 cup: 188 calories 13g fat
381mg cholesterol 248mg sodium
4g carbohydrate (3g sugars, 1g fiber) 14g protein.

51 Red Pepper Egg-In-A-Hole

Total Time: 20 mins
Servings 4 servings

Ingredients

- olive oil spray
- 1 bell pepper cut into 4 1/2" thick rings
- 4 large eggs
- salt and fresh pepper

Instructions

- In a large nonstick skillet, heat on medium heat.
- When hot, spray olive oil spray, add pepper and let it cook a minute, then add egg into the center of the pepper.
- Season with salt and pepper and cook until the egg whites are mostly set but the yolks are still runny, 2-3 minutes.
- Gently flip and cook 1 more minute for over easy, longer if you like them over well.

Nutrition Info

Serving: 1egg

Calories: 80kcal

Carbohydrates: 1.5g

Protein: 6.5g

Fat: 5g

Polyunsaturated Fat: 0g

Monounsaturated Fat

0g, Trans Fat: 0g

Potassium: 0mg

Fiber: 0.5g

52 Corned Beef and Cabbage

A simple way to prepare this classic Irish dish. Top it with horseradish cream or mustard and serve it with a side of creamy cauliflower puree as a low carb alternative to potatoes.

Prep Time: 5 mins

Cook Time: 3 hrs

Total Time: 3 hrs

Servings 4 servings

Ingredients

- 2.5 lbs corned beef brisket in brine, fat trimmed off
- 1 cup baby carrots, peeled
- 1 small head cabbage, cut into 4 wedges
- 2 bay leaves

For the Horseradish Cream (Optional)

- 1 tbsp prepared grated horseradish
- 1/4 cup fat free sour cream, full fat for Keto
- 1/4 tsp dijon mustard
- salt and pepper

Instructions

- In a large pot, place brisket, bay leaves and enough water to cover.
- Simmer, covered for about an hour per pound.
- When meat is tender add carrots.
- Boil for about 10 minutes, then add cabbage.
- Cook another 15- 20 minutes, until tender.
- Remove the meat and place on a cutting board.
- Slice the meat across the grain into thin slices.
- Serve with vegetables and ladle some broth on top.

Nutrition Info

Serving: 1/4 of meat and veggies

Calories: 292.5kcal

Carbohydrates: 20.5g

Protein: 19.3g

Fat: 16.1g

Saturated Fat: 5.5g

Polyunsaturated Fat: 0g

Monounsaturated Fat: 0g

Trans Fat: 0g

Cholesterol: 83mg

Sodium: 960mg

Potassium: 0mg

Fiber: 8.3g

Sugar: 3g

53 Homemade Chicken Broth

What's better than coming home to homemade chicken stock and cleaning out your refrigerator at the same time. Simply throw all the ingredients into the Slow Cooker the night before, turn it on in the morning and come home to a splendid broth.

Prep Time: 10 mins

Ingredients

- 3 chicken breast halves
- 1 onion, quartered
- 1 to mato, quartered
- 1 cup carrots
- 2 celery stalks
- 2 cloves garlic
- 2-3 sprigs thyme
- 3 bay leaves
- fresh herbs like cilantro or parsley, I used cilantro
- whole peppercorns
- kosher salt

Instructions

- Place all ingredients into crock pot and fill with water.
- Cover and cook on high for 4 hours or low for 8 hours.
- When it's done, throw out all the vegetables, strain the liquid and remove the chicken for other recipes, like chicken salad, or anything that calls for shredded chicken.
- If you're not using the stock right away you can store it in containers and refrigerate for up to 2 days or freeze for several months.
- When the stock is chilled, the fat will rise to the top and harden and you can easily remove it.

Nutrition Info

Calories: 10kcal

Carbohydrates: 0g

Protein: 1g, Fat: 0g

Saturated Fat: 0g

Polyunsaturated Fat: 0g

Monounsaturated Fat: 0g

54 Garlic Shrimp

Servings 3 servings

Ingredients

- 1 lb large shrimp, peeled and deveined (weight after you peel them)
- 6 cloves garlic, sliced thin
- 1 tbsp Spanish olive oil
- crushed red pepper flakes
- pinch paprika
- salt
- 1/4 cup chopped fresh herbs like cilantro or parsley
- Lime wedges for serving

Instructions

- In a large skillet, heat oil on medium heat and add the garlic and red pepper flakes.
- Sauté until golden, about 2 minutes being careful not to burn.
- Add shrimp and season with salt and paprika.
- Cook 2-3 minutes until shrimp is cooked through.
- Do not overcook or it will become tough and chewy.
- Add chopped fresh herbs and divide equally in 3 plates.

Nutrition Info

Calories: 210.5kcal   Carbohydrates: 3.6g

Protein: 31.2g   Fat: 7.2g

Polyunsaturated Fat: 0g   Monounsaturated Fat: 0g

Trans Fat: 0g   Potassium: 0mg

55 Easy Low-Carb Cauliflower Mac 'n Cheese

This low-carb keto cauliflower mac 'n cheese is a wonderful alternative to the traditional version, and a great vegetarian main dish as well.

Prep 15 m
Cook 25 m
Ready In 40 m

Ingredients

- 1 head cauliflower, cut into florets
- 1 teaspoon salt
- 1 teaspoon mixed herbs
- 1/2 teaspoon ground black pepper
- 3 tablespoons olive oil
- 1 cup shredded Cheddar cheese
- 1/2 cup heavy whipping cream
- 1 tablespoon ghee (clarified butter)
- 1 pinch ground nutmeg
- 3 tablespoons grated Parmesan cheese

Instructions

- Preheat oven to 450 degrees F (230 degrees C). Line a baking sheet with aluminum foil.
- Arrange cauliflower on the prepared baking sheet. Sprinkle with salt, mixed herbs, and pepper. Drizzle with olive oil; toss until well coated.

- Roast in the preheated oven until crisp, 10 to 15 minutes. Place in an 8-inch baking dish.
- Combine Cheddar cheese, heavy cream, ghee, and nutmeg in a saucepan over medium heat; simmer until bubbly, about 5 minutes. Pour over cauliflower; mix well. Sprinkle Parmesan cheese on top.
- Bake in the preheated oven until golden, about 10 minutes.

Nutrition Info

Per Serving: 389 calories	35 g fat
9.5 g carbohydrates	12 g protein
82 mg cholesterol	869 mg sodium

56 Cheesy Broccoli and Chicken Casserole

Prep: 15 mins
Cook: 1 hr
Total: 1 hr 25 mins
Additional: 10 mins
Servings: 10

Ingredients

2 heads broccoli, cut into florets

- 1 large rotisserie chicken, meat pulled and shredded
- 1 cup mayonnaise
- 1/2 cup heavy whipping cream
- 1 tablespoon chicken soup base
- 1 tablespoon dried dill weed

- 1 teaspoon ground black pepper
- 2 cups shredded Cheddar cheese
- cooking spray

Instructions

- Preheat oven to 350 degrees F (175 degrees C).
- Place broccoli florets in a 9x13-inch baking dish. Layer shredded chicken on top; press down onto broccoli.
- Combine mayonnaise, heavy cream, chicken soup base, dill, and pepper in a bowl; mix well. Spread evenly over chicken and top with Cheddar cheese. Grease a piece of aluminum foil with cooking spray and cover baking dish with greased-side down.
- Bake covered in the preheated oven, about 45 minutes. Remove aluminum foil and bake until golden brown, about 15 minutes. Remove from oven and let stand for 10 to 20 minutes before serving.

Nutrition Info

357 calories   31.8 g total fat
69 mg cholesterol   520 mg sodium. 6 g carbohydrates
13.4 g protein

57 Garlic and Herb Mashed Cauliflower

Prep/Cook Time: 30 min
4 servings

Ingredients

- 2 heads cauliflower
- 2 tablespoons olive oil
- 3 cloves garlic, chopped
- ½ cup sour cream (115 g)
- ½ cup fresh chives, chopped (20 g)
- ¼ cup fresh parsley (10 g)
- 1 teaspoon salt
- 1 teaspoon pepper

Instructions

- Wrap cauliflower in a clean dish towel, then turn it upside down and bang it against the surface of your counter until you feel the cauliflower crack (be sure to rotate to break it up on all sides).
- Pull florets off of stem and break the bigger florets into smaller pieces.
- Bring a large pot of water to boil over high heat.
- Add the cauliflower pieces to the pot and boil, covered, for 15-18 minutes.
- Drain the cauliflower.
- Mash the cauliflower with a fork until smooth.
- Mix in remaining ingredients. Allow to cool for 5 minutes.
- Enjoy!

Nutrition Info

Calories 197   Fat 12g

Carbs 19g   Fiber 7g

Sugar 7g   Protein 7g

58 Bolognese Sauce

Bolognese sauce is a ground beef ragú made with pancetta, onions, carrots, celery, tomatoes, wine, and cream. I decided to tweak my recipe to make this lighter version by using lean chopped beef, reducing the butter and using half and half instead of heavy cream.

Total Time: 2 hrs

Servings 16 servings

Ingredients

- 4 oz pancetta, chopped (or center cut bacon)
- 1 tbsp butter
- 1 small onion, chopped
- 1/2 cup celery, minced
- 1/2 cup carrots, minced
- 1 lb 95% lean ground beef
- 1/4 cup white wine
- 2 - 28 oz cans crushed tomatoes, I love Tuttorosso
- 1 bay leaf
- salt and fresh pepper
- 1/4 cup chopped fresh parsley
- 1/2 cup half & half

Instructions

- In a deep heavy saute pan, sauté pancetta until fat melts.
- Add butter, onions, celery and carrots and cook on medium-low heat until soft, about 5 minutes.
- Increase flame to medium-high, add meat, season with salt and pepper and sauté until browned.
- Add wine, cook until it reduces down, about 3-4 minutes.
- Add tomatoes and bay leaf. Simmer covered on low, at least 1-1/2 to 2 hours, stirring occasionally.
- Add half & half and parsley, cook 2 minutes longer.

Nutrition Info

Serving: 1/2 cup

Calories: 120kcal

Carbohydrates: 8g

Protein: 7.5g

Fat: 5g, Saturated Fat: 3g

Cholesterol: 77.5mg

Sodium: 335mg

Sugar: 4g

59 Gazpacho

2 servings

Ingredients

- 2 large tomatoes, peeled
- 1/2 medium cucumber, peeled and seeded
- 1/4 red bell pepper
- 1 garlic clove
- 1 tsp red wine vinegar
- 2 tsp extra virgin olive oil

- kosher salt and fresh black pepper to taste
- 2 tbsp chopped red onion

Instructions

- Place tomatoes, cucumber, bell pepper, garlic, salt, pepper and vinegar in the blender until smooth.
- Chill in refrigerator 1/2 hour.
- Pour into two large bowls and top with 1 tsp olive oil in each bowl, chopped red onion, salt and pepper plus toppings (shaved parmesan or avocado if using).
- Serve with good crusty bread.

Nutrition Info

Serving: 1bowl

Calories: 82.1kcal

Carbohydrates: 9.2g

Protein: 1.7g

Fat: 5.1g

60 Caveman Chili

Prep/Cook Time: 6 h 35 m

8 servings

Ingredients

- 2 pounds ground pork
- 8 thick slices bacon, chopped
- 1 (14.5 ounce) can diced tomatoes, drained
- 1 onion, chopped
- 3 small green bell peppers, chopped

- 1 (6 ounce) can tomato paste
- 1 (1.25 ounce) package chili seasoning (such as McCormick)
- 1 pinch garlic powder, or more to taste
- 1 pinch onion powder, or more to taste
- salt and ground black pepper to taste
- 1 pinch ground cayenne pepper, or more to taste

Instructions

- Place pork in a skillet over medium heat; season with salt and pepper. Cook and stir until browned and crumbly, 5 to 7 minutes. Drain and discard grease. Transfer pork to a slow cooker.
- Place bacon in the hot skillet and cook over medium-high heat until evenly browned, about 10 minutes. Drain and discard grease. Transfer bacon to the slow cooker.
- Combine drained tomatoes, onion, green bell pepper, and tomato paste into the slow cooker. Add seasoning packet, garlic powder, onion powder, and salt, pepper, cayenne pepper; stir to combine.
- Cook on Low until flavors have combined, about 6 hours.

Nutrition Info

357 calories	22 g fat
12.2 g carbohydrates	27.4 g protein
87 mg cholesterol	1031 mg sodium

61 Keto Cheesecake Cupcakes

Prep/Cook Time: 8 h 25 m   12 servings

Ingredients

- 1/2 cup almond meal
- 1/4 cup butter, melted
- 2 (8 ounce) packages cream cheese, softened
- 2 eggs
- 3/4 cup granular no-calorie sucralose sweetener (such as Splenda)
- 1 teaspoon vanilla extract

Instructions

- Preheat oven to 350 degrees F (175 degrees C). Line 12 muffin cups with paper liners.
- Mix almond meal and butter together in a bowl; spoon into the bottoms of the paper liners and press into a flat crust.
- Beat cream cheese, eggs, sweetener, and vanilla extract together in a bowl with an electric mixer set to medium until smooth; spoon over the crust layer in the paper liners.
- Bake in the preheated oven until the cream cheese mixture is nearly set in the middle, 15 to 17 minutes.
- Let cupcakes cool at room temperature until cool enough to handle. Refrigerate 8 hours to overnight before serving.

Nutrition Info

Per Serving: 204 calories   20 g fat; 2.1 g carbohydrates
4.9 g protein   82 mg cholesterol
151 mg sodium

62 Keto Beef Egg Roll Slaw

Prep/Cook Time: 30 m
6 servings

Ingredients

- 2 tablespoons sesame oil
- 1/2 cup diced onion
- 5 green onions, chopped, white and green parts separated
- 3 cloves garlic, minced
- 1 1/2 pounds ground beef
- 1 tablespoon chili-garlic sauce (such as sriracha)
- 1/2 teaspoon ground ginger
- sea salt to taste
- ground black pepper to taste
- 1 (14 ounce) package coleslaw mix
- 3 tablespoons soy sauce
- 1 tablespoon apple cider vinegar

Instructions

- Heat oil in a large skillet over medium-high heat. Add diced onion, white parts of the green onions, and garlic. Saute until onions are translucent and garlic is fragrant, about 5 minutes. Add ground beef, sriracha, ginger, salt, and black pepper. Saute until beef is browned and crumbly, about 5 minutes.
- Stir coleslaw mix, soy sauce, and cider vinegar into the beef mixture. Saute until coleslaw is tender, about 4 minutes more. Top with the rest of the green onions.

Nutrition Info

Per Serving: 350 calories   24 g fat

12 g carbohydrates   20.6 g protein

75 mg cholesterol   694 mg sodium

63 Creamy Keto Taco Soup with Ground Beef

This keto-friendly, low-carb, Southwestern taco soup is full of ground beef, cream cheese, heavy cream, and spices. Freezing is not recommended."

Prep/Cook Time: 30 m

8 servings

288 cals

Ingredients

- 1 pound ground beef
- 1/2 cup chopped onion
- 2 cloves garlic, minced
- 1 tablespoon ground cumin
- 1 teaspoon chili powder
- 1 (8 ounce) package cream cheese, softened
- 2 (14.5 ounce) cans beef broth
- 2 (10 ounce) cans diced tomatoes and green chiles (such as RO*TEL)
- 1/2 cup heavy cream
- 2 teaspoons salt, or to taste

Instructions

- Combine ground beef with onion and garlic in a large soup pot over medium-high heat. Cook and stir until beef is browned and crumbly, 5 to 7 minutes. Drain and discard grease. Add cumin and chili powder; cook 2 minutes more.
- Drop cream cheese into the pot by bits and mash it into the beef with a big spoon until no white spots remain, 3 to 5 minutes. Stir in broth, diced tomatoes, heavy cream, and salt. Cook until heated through, about 10 minutes more.

Nutrition Info

Per Serving: 288 calories   24 g fat; 5.4 g carbohydrates

13.4 g protein   85 mg cholesterol

1310 mg sodium.

64 Ketogenic Bread

Make sure when you make this recipe, that you place baking paper in the tray while baking. The first time I did this was without baking paper. Trust me, this is not what you want to be scraping out of the tin. Finding it hard to give up carbohydrates? This keto bread makes the switch much easier, so you can still have sandwiches and toast."

Prep/Cook Time: 55 m

8 servings

Ingredients

- 7 eggs
- 1/2 cup butter, melted
- 2 tablespoons coconut oil
- 2 cups almond flour
- 1 teaspoon baking powder
- 1/2 teaspoon xanthan gum
- 1/2 teaspoon salt

Instructions

- Preheat oven to 350 degrees F (175 degrees C). Line a loaf pan with parchment paper.
- Beat eggs in a bowl using an electric mixer on high until frothy, 1 to 2 minutes. Add butter and coconut oil; continue beating until smooth. Mix almond flour, baking powder, xanthan gum, and salt into egg mixture until dough is well mixed and very thick; transfer to the prepared loaf pan.
- Bake in the preheated oven until a skewer inserted in the center comes out clean, about 45 minutes.

Nutrition Info

Per Serving: 377 calories   34.7 g fat

7.5 g carbohydrates   12.2 g protein

193 mg cholesterol   357 mg sodium

65 Instant Pot Spicy Butternut Squash Soup

This quick and easy butternut squash soup is so flavorful with ginger and brown sugar; and it only takes a few minutes in your Instant Pot

Prep/Cook Time: 1 h
6 servings

Ingredients

- 1 tablespoon olive oil
- 1 onion, diced
- 2 cloves garlic
- 1 pound butternut squash - peeled, seeded, and cut into 1-inch pieces
- 5 cups vegetable broth
- 1 tablespoon brown sugar
- 1 teaspoon salt
- 1/2 teaspoon ground black pepper
- 1/2 teaspoon ground ginger
- 1/2 teaspoon curry powder (optional)
- 1 cup heavy whipping cream

Instructions

- Turn on a multi-functional pressure cooker (such as Instant Pot(R)) and select Saute function. Heat olive oil and add onion; cook until translucent, about 7 minutes. Add garlic and cook for 1 minute more.
- Combine butternut squash, vegetable broth, brown sugar, salt, ground black pepper, ginger, and curry powder in the pot. Close

and lock the lid. Select high pressure according to manufacturer's instructions; set timer for 10 minutes. Allow 10 to 15 minutes for pressure to build.

- Release pressure carefully using the quick-release method according to manufacturer's instructions, about 5 minutes. Unlock and remove lid. Blend with an immersion blender until creamy.
- Stir in heavy whipping cream.

Nutrition Info

Per Serving: 235 calories

17.5 g fat

18.7 g carbohydrates

2.7 g protein

54 mg cholesterol

791 mg sodium

66 Ultimate Low-Carb Zucchini Lasagna

Zucchini slices step in for pasta in this low-carb and gluten-free beef lasagna that is delicious and satisfying; such a crowd pleaser!"

Prep/Cook Time: 1 h 20 m   6 servings

Ingredients

- cooking spray
- 1 1/2 large zucchinis, thinly sliced lengthwise
- 1 tablespoon olive oil
- 1 pound ground beef
- 1 1/2 cups low-carb marinara sauce
- 2 teaspoons salt, divided
- 1 teaspoon dried oregano

- 1/2 teaspoon ground black pepper
- 1 (8 ounce) container ricotta cheese
- 1 egg
- 1/2 teaspoon ground nutmeg
- 2 cups shredded mozzarella cheese, divided
- 1/4 cup grated Parmesan cheese

Instructions

- Preheat oven to 375 degrees F (190 degrees C). Grease an 8-inch baking dish with cooking spray.
- Pat dry zucchini slices with a paper towel to get rid of excess moisture.
- Heat olive oil in a saucepan over medium-high heat. Add ground beef; cook until browned, 5 to 8 minutes. Add marinara sauce, 1 teaspoon salt, oregano, and pepper; simmer for 10 minutes.
- Combine remaining 1 teaspoon salt, ricotta cheese, egg, and nutmeg in a bowl; mix well.
- Make 1 layer of zucchini slices in the prepared baking dish. Cover with 1/2 of the sauce. Add another layer of zucchini slices. Spread ricotta mixture on top. Sprinkle with 1 cup mozzarella cheese. Add another layer of zucchini slices; cover with the remaining sauce and top with 1 cup mozzarella cheese and Parmesan cheese. Cover baking dish with aluminum foil.
- Bake in the preheated oven for 30 minutes. Remove aluminum foil and bake until top is golden, about 15 minutes more.

Nutrition Info

Per Serving: 424 calories

14.9 g carbohydrates

117 mg cholesterol

26.8 g fat

30.4 g protein

1427 mg sodium.

129

67 Keto Brownies

Get your chocolate fix with these yummy low-carb brownies.

Prep/Cook Time: 40 m
12 servings

Ingredients

- 3/4 cup cocoa powder
- 1/2 teaspoon baking soda
- 2/3 cup coconut oil, divided
- 1/2 cup boiling water
- 1 cup stevia sugar substitute (such as Truvia)
- 2 eggs
- 1 1/3 cups almond flour
- 1 teaspoon vanilla extract
- 1/4 teaspoon salt

Instructions

- Preheat oven to 350 degrees F (175 degrees C). Lightly grease an 8-inch square pan with coconut oil.
- Whisk cocoa powder and baking soda together in a bowl. Add 1/3 cup coconut oil and boiling water; mix until well blended. Add remaining 1/3 cup coconut oil, stevia, and eggs; blend well. Fold almond flour, vanilla extract, and salt into the batter.
- Pour batter into the greased pan.
- Bake in the preheated oven until top is dry and edges have started to pull away from the sides of the pan, 30 to 40 minutes. Let cool before cutting into 12 squares.

Nutrition Info

Per Serving: 222 calories   20.5 g fat
17.5 g carbohydrates   5 g protein
31 mg cholesterol   114 mg sodium.

68 Keto Chicken Parmesan

A delicious keto-friendly chicken Parmesan. Enjoy a classic Italian dish, and keep your macros in check!

Prep/Cook Time: 28 m
2 servings

Ingredients

- 1 (8 ounce) skinless, boneless chicken breast
- 1 egg
- 1 tablespoon heavy whipping cream
- 1 1/2 ounces pork rinds, crushed
- 1 ounce grated Parmesan cheese
- 1/2 teaspoon salt
- 1/2 teaspoon garlic powder
- 1/2 teaspoon red pepper flakes (optional)
- 1/2 teaspoon ground black pepper
- 1/2 teaspoon Italian seasoning
- 1/2 cup jarred tomato sauce (such as Rao's)
- 1/4 cup shredded mozzarella cheese
- 1 tablespoon ghee (clarified butter)

Instructions

- Set oven rack about 6 inches from the heat source and preheat the oven's broiler.
- Slice chicken breast through the middle horizontally from one side to within 1/2 inch of the other side. Open the two sides and spread them out like an open book. Pound chicken flat until about 1/2-inch thick.
- Beat egg and cream together in a bowl.
- Combine crushed pork rinds, Parmesan cheese, salt, garlic powder, red pepper flakes, ground black pepper, and Italian seasoning in bowl; transfer breading to a plate.
- Dip chicken into egg mixture; coat completely. Press chicken into breading; thickly coat both sides.
- Heat a skillet over medium-high heat; add ghee. Place chicken in the pan; cook until no longer pink in the center and the juices run clear, about 3 minutes per side. An instant-read thermometer inserted into the center should read at least 165 degrees F (74 degrees C). Be careful to keep breading in place.
- Transfer chicken to a baking sheet. Cover with tomato sauce; top with mozzarella cheese.
- Broil until cheese is bubbling and barely browned, about 2 minutes.

Nutrition Info

Per Serving: 442 calories	25.3 g fat
5.8 g carbohydrates	46.5 g protein
217 mg cholesterol	1605 mg sodium

69 Creamy Keto Cauliflower Risotto

Mushrooms, cauliflower, heavy cream, and Parmesan cheese combine in this creamy low-carb risotto, perfect as a side dish or even as a main dish.

Prep/Cook Time: 29 m
4 servings

Ingredients

- 1/4 cup ghee
- 1/2 onion, finely chopped
- 1 clove garlic, minced
- 1 head cauliflower, grated
- 1 cup sliced fresh mushrooms
- 1/2 cup heavy whipping cream
- 1 cup grated Parmesan cheese
- 1/2 teaspoon salt
- 1/4 teaspoon ground black pepper
- 1/4 teaspoon ground nutmeg

Instructions

- Melt ghee in a skillet over medium heat. Add onion and garlic; cook until tender, about 3 minutes. Stir in grated cauliflower; cook for 3 minutes more. Add mushrooms and cook until tender, about 3 minutes.

- Stir heavy cream, Parmesan cheese, salt, pepper, and nutmeg into the skillet; cook over medium heat until creamy, 5 to 7 minutes.

Nutrition Info

Per Serving: 350 calories   29.8 g fat

11.8 g carbohydrates   12.1 g protein

91 mg cholesterol   653 mg sodium

70 Chocolate-Peanut Butter Keto Cups

This is a modification of a recipe for a peanut butter cup-style fat-bomb I found online. Store in the fridge or freezer. When hungry or needing a fat bomb (if you are on keto), eat one.

Prep/Cook Time: 1 h 18 m   12 servings

Ingredients

- 1 cup coconut oil
- 1/2 cup natural peanut butter
- 2 tablespoons heavy cream
- 1 tablespoon cocoa powder
- 1 teaspoon liquid stevia
- 1/4 teaspoon vanilla extract
- 1/4 teaspoon kosher salt
- 1 ounce chopped roasted salted peanuts

Instructions

- Melt coconut oil in a saucepan over low heat, 3 to 5 minutes. Stir in peanut butter until smooth. Whisk in heavy cream, cocoa powder, liquid stevia, vanilla extract, and salt.
- Pour chocolate-peanut butter mixture into 12 silicone muffin molds. Sprinkle peanuts evenly on top. Place molds on a baking sheet.
- Freeze chocolate-peanut butter mixture until firm, at least 1 hour. Unmold chocolate-peanut cups and transfer to a resealable plastic bag or airtight container.

Nutrition Info

Per Serving: 246 calories   26 g fat

3.3 g carbohydrates   3.4 g protein

3 mg cholesterol   89 mg sodium

71 Grain-Free Butter Bread

Prep/Cook Time: 1 h

8 servings

Ingredients

- 6 eggs
- 1 1/2 cups finely ground almond flour
- 1 teaspoon fine salt
- 2 teaspoons baking powder
- 1/4 cup melted butter
- 1/8 teaspoon cream of tartar

Instructions

- Separate eggs. Crack each egg into your hand and let the whites run into a bowl. Place yolks in a second bowl.
- Preheat the oven to 375 degrees F (190 degrees C). Butter a loaf pan and line the bottom with parchment paper.
- Place almond flour in a food processor. Add salt, baking powder, and egg yolks. Pour in melted butter. Pulse, scraping down the sides once or twice, until mixture comes together.
- Sprinkle cream of tartar into the egg whites. Whisk until soft peaks form. Transfer about 1/3 of the mixture into the food processor. Pulse on and off, scraping mixture down with a spatula as needed, until well blended. Scrape mixture into the bowl with the egg whites. Fold together until well combined but still airy. Pour batter into the prepared loaf pan.
- Bake in the preheated oven until golden brown and a toothpick inserted into the center comes out clean, about 30 minutes.
- Run a thin knife along the edge bread and let rest for 10 minutes. Turn bread out onto a wire rack and cool to room temperature before slicing.

Nutrition Info

Per Serving: 241 calories   21 g fat

5.6 g carbohydrates   9.7 g protein

155 mg cholesterol   506 mg sodium

72 Garlic Tuscan Chicken

This is a great quick keto-friendly meal. Serve over pasta if desired."

Prep/Cook Time: 25 m
4 servings

Ingredients

- 2 tablespoons olive oil
- 1 1/2 pounds skinless, boneless chicken breasts, thinly sliced
- 1 cup heavy cream
- 1/2 cup chicken broth
- 1/2 cup grated Parmesan cheese
- 1 teaspoon garlic powder
- 1 teaspoon Italian seasoning
- 1 cup spinach, chopped
- 1/2 cup chopped sun-dried tomatoes

Instructions

- Heat olive oil in a large skillet over medium-high heat. Cook chicken until browned and no longer pink in the center, 3 to 5 minutes per side. Remove chicken and set aside on a plate.
- Add heavy cream, chicken broth, Parmesan cheese, garlic powder, and Italian seasoning to the skillet. Whisk sauce over medium-high heat until starting to thicken, about 5 minutes. Add spinach and sun-dried tomatoes; simmer until spinach starts to wilt, about 1 minute. Return chicken to the skillet and cook until heated through, 2 to 3 minutes.

Nutrition Info

Per Serving: 505 calories

35.4 g fat

7 g carbohydrates

39.6 g protein

179 mg cholesterol

540 mg sodium

73 Low-Carb Almond Cinnamon Butter Cookies

Prep/Cook Time: 23 m

12 servings

Ingredients

- 2 cups blanched almond flour
- 1/2 cup butter, softened
- 1 egg
- 1/2 cup low-calorie natural sweetener (such as Swerve)
- 1 teaspoon sugar-free vanilla extract
- 1 teaspoon ground cinnamon

Instructions

- Preheat oven to 350 degrees F (175 degrees C). Line a baking sheet with parchment paper.
- Combine almond flour, butter, egg, sweetener, vanilla extract, and cinnamon in a bowl; mix until well combined.
- Roll dough into 1-inch balls. Place on the prepared baking sheet and press down with a fork twice in a criss-cross pattern.
- Bake in the the preheated oven until edges are golden, 12 to 15 minutes. Cool on the baking sheet for 1 minute before removing to a wire rack to cool completely.

Nutrition Info

Per Serving: 196 calories

12.7 g carbohydrates

36 mg cholesterol

18.4 g fat

5 g protein

60 mg sodium

74 Simple Cauliflower Keto Casserole

Cauliflower in a creamy cheese sauce is a perfect keto recipe and delicious to boot! Make sure you season well with salt and pepper (nutmeg tastes great as well) otherwise it will taste too bland.

Prep/Cook Time: 45 m   2 servings

Ingredients

- 1/2 head cauliflower florets
- 1 cup shredded Cheddar cheese
- 1/2 cup heavy cream
- 1 pinch salt and freshly ground black pepper to taste

Instructions

- Preheat the oven to 400 degrees F (200 degrees C).
- Bring a large pot of slightly salted water to a boil and cook cauliflower until tender but firm to the bite, about 10 minutes. Drain.
- Combine Cheddar cheese, cream, salt, and pepper in a large bowl. Arrange cauliflower in a casserole dish and cover with cheese mixture.
- Bake in the preheated oven until cheese is bubbly and golden brown, about 25 minutes.

Nutrition Info

Per Serving: 469 calories   40.9 g fat

10 g carbohydrates   18.1 g protein

141 mg cholesterol   494 mg sodium

75 Roasted Brussels Sprouts

Try these crispy roasted Brussels sprouts made in just 5 minutes in your Instant Pot; they're a quick and easy low-carb side dish that's family-friendly.

Prep/Cook Time: 26 m

4 servings

Ingredients

- 2 tablespoons olive oil
- 1 onion, chopped
- 1 pound whole Brussels sprouts
- 1 teaspoon salt
- 1/2 teaspoon ground black pepper
- 1/2 cup vegetable broth

Instructions

- Turn on a multi-functional pressure cooker (such as Instant Pot(R)) and select Saute function. Heat olive oil and cook onion until translucent, about 2 minutes. Add Brussels sprouts and cook for 1 minute more. Sprinkle with salt and pepper; pour vegetable broth over Brussels sprouts. Close and lock the lid.

Select high pressure according to manufacturer's instructions; set timer for 3 minutes. Allow 10 to 15 minutes for pressure to build.

- Release pressure carefully using the quick-release method according to manufacturer's instructions, about 5 minutes. Unlock and remove lid.

Nutrition Info

Per Serving: 136 calories   7.2 g fat
16.3 g carbohydrates   4.6 g protein
0 mg cholesterol   670 mg sodium

76 Salsa Picante Roja

This spicy red salsa is made with fresh tomatoes, roasted jalapeño, garlic and cilantro, pureed in a blender then simmered until the tomatoes deepen in color. Serve with your favorite baked chips and Sinless Margaritas!

Prep Time: 10 mins
Cook Time: 20 mins
Total Time: 30 mins
Servings 6 servings

Ingredients

- 3 medium tomatoes, cored and quartered
- 1 jalapeño, stem removed and roasted
- 3-4 small cloves garlic

- 2 tbsp cilantro
- 3-4 tbsp water
- 1 tsp olive oil
- salt to taste

Instructions

- In a blender, add tomatoes, jalapeño, garlic, cilantro and water and pulse a few times until completely smooth.
- Add oil to a deep skillet, then pour in tomatoes.
- Season with salt and simmer uncovered stirring occasionally, 20 to 25 minutes.
- Depending on the size of your tomatoes, makes about 1 1/2 cups. You can refrigerate a few days or freeze the rest.

Nutrition Info

Serving: 1/4 cup

Calories: 22.5kcal

Carbohydrates: 3.5g

Protein: 0.5g, Fat: 1g

Saturated Fat: 0g

Polyunsaturated Fat: 0g

Monounsaturated Fat: 0g

Trans Fat: 0g

77 Low Fat Red Wine Tomato Vinaigrette

Prep/Cook Time: 30 mins
8 servings

Ingredients

- 1 medium red ripe tomato
- 1 clove crushed garlic
- 1 tbsp red wine vinegar
- 3 tbsp extra virgin olive oil
- 1 tsp dijon mustard
- 1 tbsp lemon juice
- 2 tbsp water
- 1/2 tsp oregano
- salt and fresh pepper to taste
- 1 tbsp minced shallot

Instructions

- Chop tomato in food processor.
- Add crushed garlic, vinegar, lemon juice, water, dijon mustard, oregano, salt and pepper.
- Pulse a few times until smooth.
- Add chopped shallot and mix well.
- Set aside a few hours to allow the flavors to blend well.

Nutrition Info

Serving: 2tbsp

Calories: 51kcal

Carbohydrates: 1.3g

Protein: 0g

Fat: 5.1g

Polyunsaturated Fat: 0g

Monounsaturated Fat: 0g

Trans Fat: 0g

Potassium: 0mg

Fiber: 0.2g

Sugar: 0.2g

78 Halibut and Shellfish Soup

A great tasting hearty seafood and shellfish soup made with halibut, littleneck clams and shrimp. Serve this with a crusty piece of bread and you have yourself a complete meal.

Prep Time: 15 mins

Cook Time: 15 mins

Total Time: 30 mins

Servings 4 servings

Ingredients

- 1 tsp olive oil
- 2 chopped shallots
- 2 cloves of garlic
- 3 medium diced tomatoes
- 4 oz dry white wine
- 1 cup clam juice
- 2 cups vegetable stock

- 3/4 lb halibut filet, skin removed cut into large pieces
- 1 lb shrimp, peeled deveined fresh shrimp
- 1 dozen littleneck clams
- pinch of saffron
- 1/4 cup fresh chopped parsley
- crusty bread for serving on the side, optional

Instructions

- Add olive oil to a large heavy pot; over medium heat sautée shallots and garlic until translucent.
- Add the tomatoes, wine, clam juice and the bone from the halibut if you have one.
- Add vegetable stock, saffron, fresh thyme and stir.
- Add the clams; cover and cook 2 minutes, add the shrimp and fish and cook and additional 3 to 5 minutes, or until the shrimp turns pink and the clams open.
- Remove bone and serve with a crusty bread to dip into the juice.

Nutrition Info

Serving: 1large bowl

Calories: 300.4kcal

Carbohydrates: 9.4g

Protein: 49.8g

Fat: 5.8g

Saturated Fat: 1g

Polyunsaturated Fat: 0g

Monounsaturated Fat: 0g

Trans Fat: 0g

Cholesterol: 220mg

Sodium: 1023.3mg

Potassium: 0mg

Fiber: 1.2g

Sugar: 1.5g

79 Grilled Tuna over Arugula with Lemon Vinaigrette

Prep/Cook Time: 20 mins
1 serving

Ingredients

- 5 oz sashimi tuna, sushi grade
- 1 tsp extra virgin olive oil
- 1 tsp fresh lemon juice
- 2 cups baby arugula
- 1 tsp capers
- kosher salt and fresh pepper

Instructions

- Season tuna with kosher salt and fresh cracked pepper.
- Place arugula and capers on a plate.
- Combine oil and lemon juice, salt and pepper.
- Heat your grill to high heat and clean grate well.
- When grill is hot, spray grate with oil to prevent sticking then place tuna on the grill; cook one minute without moving.
- Turn over and cook an additional minute; remove from heat and set aside on a plate.
- Slice tuna on the diagonal and place on top of salad.
- Top with lemon vinaigrette and eat immediately.

Nutrition Info

Serving: 5oz tuna and salad	Calories: 297.8kcal
Carbohydrates: 3.8g	Protein: 35.4g
Fat: 15.5g	Polyunsaturated Fat: 0g
Monounsaturated Fat: 0g	Trans Fat: 0g
Sodium: 326.3mg	Potassium: 0mg
Fiber: 1.6g	Sugar: 1.8g

80 Fluffy Keto Pancakes

These fluffy, tasty pancakes are super easy. Serve with plenty of butter and your favorite sugar-free syrup.

Prep/Cook Time: 15 m
4 servings

Ingredients

- 1 cup almond flour
- 1/4 cup coconut flour
- 2 tablespoons low-calorie natural sweetener (such as Swerve)
- 1 teaspoon salt
- 1 teaspoon baking powder
- 1/2 teaspoon ground cinnamon (optional)
- 6 eggs, at room temperature
- 1/4 cup heavy whipping cream, at room temperature
- 2 tablespoons butter, melted
- 1 teaspoon vanilla extract

Instructions

- Mix almond flour, coconut flour, sweetener, salt, baking powder, and cinnamon together in a bowl. Whisk in eggs, heavy cream, butter, and vanilla extract slowly until batter is just blended.
- Heat a lightly oiled griddle over medium-high heat. Drop batter by large spoonfuls onto the griddle and cook until bubbles form and the edges are dry, 3 to 4 minutes. Flip and cook until browned on the other side, 2 to 3 minutes. Repeat with remaining batter.

Nutrition Info

Per Serving: 383 calories

33.2 g fat

13.4 g carbohydrates

15.3 g protein

281 mg cholesterol

842 mg sodium

81 Chilled Calamari Salad with Lemon and Parsley

Prep/Cook Time: 1 hour
4 servings

Ingredients

- 1/4 cup red onion, minced
- 1/2 cup celery, chopped
- 1/2 cup roasted red peppers, chopped
- 1/4 cup fresh parsley, minced (no stems)
- 1 clove garlic, sliced
- 1 1/2 lemons
- 1 1/4 tsp red wine vinegar

- salt and fresh pepper to taste
- 1 lb fresh squid, tube and tentacles cleaned

Instructions

- Rinse squid and slice tubes into 1/2 inch rings.
- Leave the tentacles whole and set aside.
- Prepare a bowl of water with ice.
- In a medium bowl combine onion, garlic, celery, red peppers, parsley, lemon juice, vinegar, salt and fresh pepper.
- Bring a medium pot filled with water and a pinch of salt to a boil.
- Add calamari all at once and cook until tender yet cooked, (I test it by tasting a ring) about 45 - 60 seconds.
- Quickly drain when cooked and add to the ice bath until cool, 4 - 5 minutes.
- Combine squid with the salad and toss well.
- Taste for salt and add additional seasoning and lemon juice if needed.
- Cover and refrigerate at least an hour.

Nutrition Info

Calories: 121.6kcal

Carbohydrates: 7.9g

Protein: 18.3g

Fat: 1.7g

Polyunsaturated Fat: 0g

Monounsaturated Fat: 0g

Trans Fat: 0g

Sodium: 66mg

Potassium: 0mg

Fiber: 0.9g

Sugar: 1.2g

82 Oven-Baked Bacon

Prep/Cook Time: 35 m

6 servings

Ingredients

- 1 (16 ounce) package bacon

Instructions

- Preheat the oven to 350 degrees F (175 degrees C). Line a baking sheet with parchment paper.
- Place bacon slices one next to the other on the prepared baking sheet.
- Bake in the preheated oven for 15 to 20 minutes. Remove from oven. Flip bacon slices with kitchen tongs and return to oven. Bake until crispy, 15 to 20 minutes more. Thinner slices will need less time, about 20 minutes total. Drain on a plate lined with paper towels.

Nutrition Info

Per Serving: 134 calories

0.4 g carbohydrates

27 mg cholesterol

10.4 g fat

9.2 g protein

574 mg sodium

83 Tuscan Pork Tenderloin

This is a very easy weeknight pork tenderloin recipe that is also keto-friendly.

Prep/Cook Time: 30 m   12 servings

Ingredients

- 4 teaspoons garlic, minced
- 2 teaspoons dried rosemary
- 2 teaspoons dried oregano
- 1 teaspoon salt
- 1 teaspoon ground black pepper
- 4 pounds pork tenderloin

Instructions

- Preheat the oven to 425 degrees F (220 degrees C).
- Combine garlic, rosemary, oregano, salt, and pepper in a small bowl. Rub spice mixture all over the pork tenderloin. Place in a baking dish.
- Bake in the preheated oven until pork is slightly pink in the center, 20 to 25 minutes. An instant-read thermometer inserted into the center should read at least 145 degrees F (63 degrees C). Remove from oven and let stand for 5 minutes before slicing.

Nutrition Info

Per Serving: 183 calories   7.3 g fat

0.7 g carbohydrates   26.9 g protein

84 mg cholesterol   251 mg sodium

84 Rebekah's Keto Egg Casserole

Egg casserole can easily be made with any breakfast meat and made ahead for an easy meal.

Prep/Cook Time: 50 m
8 servings

Ingredients

- 1 (8 ounce) package breakfast sausage
- 12 eggs
- 1 (8 ounce) package shredded Cheddar cheese
- 3/4 cup heavy whipping cream
- 1 tablespoon minced onion
- 2 teaspoons dry mustard
- 1 teaspoon dried oregano
- salt and ground black pepper to taste

Instructions

- Preheat oven to 350 degrees F (175 degrees C).
- Heat a large skillet over medium-high heat. Cook sausage, breaking it apart with a wooden spoon, until browned and crumbly, 5 to 7 minutes. Spread over the bottom of a 9x13-inch casserole dish.
- Mix eggs, Cheddar cheese, cream, onion, mustard, oregano, salt, and pepper together in a bowl. Pour mixture over the sausage.
- Bake in the preheated oven until firm and cooked through, 30 to 40 minutes.

Nutrition Info

Per Serving: 374 calories

2.2 g carbohydrates

355 mg cholesterol

31.4 g fat

21 g protein

559 mg sodium

85 Lemon Rotisserie Chicken

This amazing recipe for Instant Pot lemon rotisserie chicken makes the most tender and moist chicken at home, perfect for a family dinner.

Prep/Cook Time: 49 m

6 servings

Ingredients

- 1 (2.5 pound) whole chicken
- 1 lemon, cut into 4 wedges
- 2 tablespoons olive oil
- 1 1/2 teaspoons salt
- 1 teaspoon garlic powder
- 1 teaspoon paprika
- 1/2 teaspoon ground black pepper
- 1 cup chicken broth

Instructions

- Rinse chicken and pat dry. Insert lemon wedges inside the cavity.
- Turn on a multi-functional pressure cooker (such as Instant Pot(R)) and select Saute function. Mix olive oil, salt, garlic

powder, paprika, and pepper in a bowl. Rub top part of chicken with 1/2 of the spice mixture. Place the chicken, breast side down, and cook until crispy, 3 to 4 minutes.

- Rub remaining spice mixture on the bottom side of the chicken. Flip chicken over with tongs and cook for 1 minute more.
- Remove chicken from the pot. Place trivet inside the pot; place chicken back in the pot, breast side down on the trivet, and pour in chicken broth. Close and lock the lid. Select high pressure according to manufacturer's instructions; set timer for 20 minutes. Allow 10 to 15 minutes for pressure to build. Release pressure using the natural-release method according to manufacturer's instructions, 10 to 40 minutes.

Nutrition Info

Per Serving: 284 calories   18.8 g fat
2.9 g carbohydrates   25.7 g protein
81 mg cholesterol   853 mg sodium

86 3-Ingredient Keto Peanut Butter Cookies

Kids will love these scrumptious low-carb keto cookies; all you need is peanut butter, vanilla extract, an egg, and some sugar substitute.

Prep/Cook Time: 23 m   12 servings

Ingredients

- 1 cup peanut butter
- 1/2 cup low-calorie natural sweetener (such as Swerve)
- 1 egg
- 1 teaspoon sugar-free vanilla extract

Instructions

- Preheat oven to 350 degrees F (175 degrees C). Line a baking sheet with parchment paper.
- Combine peanut butter, sweetener, egg, and vanilla extract in a bowl; mix well until a dough is formed.
- Roll dough into 1-inch balls. Place on the prepared baking sheet and press down twice with a fork in a criss-cross pattern.
- Bake in the the preheated oven until edges are golden, 12 to 15 minutes. Cool on the baking sheet for 1 minute before removing to a wire rack to cool completely.

Nutrition Info

Per Serving: 133 calories   11.2 g fat
12.4 g carbohydrates   5.9 g protein
16 mg cholesterol   105 mg sodium

87 Quick and Easy Parmesan Zucchini Fries

Zucchinis, Parmesan cheese, garlic, and paprika make these ultimate zucchini fries, that are so easy to make, and carb-conscious as well!

Prep/Cook Time: 45 m   4 servings

Ingredients

- cooking spray
- 2 eggs
- 3/4 cup grated Parmesan cheese
- 1 tablespoon dried mixed herbs
- 1 1/2 teaspoons garlic powder
- 1 teaspoon paprika
- 1/2 teaspoon ground black pepper
- 2 pounds zucchinis, cut into 1/2-inch French fry strips

Instructions

- Preheat oven to 425 degrees F (220 degrees C). Line a baking sheet with aluminum foil and spray with cooking spray.
- Whisk eggs in a shallow bowl. Combine Parmesan cheese, mixed herbs, garlic powder, paprika, and pepper in a separate shallow bowl; mix well.
- Dip zucchini fries into beaten eggs, in batches; shake to remove excess, and roll in Parmesan mixture until fully coated. Place on the prepared baking sheet.
- Bake in the preheated oven, turning once, until golden and crispy, 30 to 35 minutes.

Nutrition Info

Per Serving: 142 calories   7.2 g fat

10.4 g carbohydrates   11.7 g protein

95 mg cholesterol   284 mg sodium

88 Cheesy Keto Biscuits

Prep/Cook Time: 40 m

9 servings

Ingredients

- 2 cups almond flour
- 1 tablespoon baking powder
- 2 1/2 cups shredded Cheddar cheese
- 4 eggs
- 1/4 cup half-and-half

Instructions

- Preheat the oven to 350 degrees F (175 degrees C). Line a baking sheet with parchment paper.
- Combine almond flour and baking powder in a large bowl. Mix in Cheddar cheese by hand. Create a small well in the middle of the bowl; add eggs and half-and-half to the center. Use a large fork, spoon, or your hands to blend in the flour mixture until a sticky batter forms.
- Drop 9 portions of batter onto the prepared baking sheet.
- Bake in the preheated oven until golden, about 20 minutes.

Nutrition Info

Per Serving: 329 calories   27.1 g fat

7.2 g carbohydrates   16.7 g protein

118 mg cholesterol   391 mg sodium

89 Keto Cinnamon Granola

Grain-free granola. Suitable for the keto (low-carb, high-fat) diet. Enjoy, try it by itself, or use as cereal.

Prep/Cook Time: 18 m

8 servings

Ingredients

- 1/2 cup coarsely chopped walnuts
- 1/2 cup coarsely chopped pecans
- 1/2 cup unsweetened shredded coconut
- 1/3 cup sliced almonds
- 1 teaspoon ground cinnamon
- 2 teaspoons granulated erythritol sweetener (such as Swerve)
- 1 (1 gram) packet granular sucrolose sweetener (such as Splenda), or more to taste (optional)
- 2 tablespoons butter, melted

Instructions

- Preheat oven to 375 degrees F (190 degrees C).
- Mix walnuts, pecans, coconut, and almonds together in a bowl.

- Stir cinnamon, erythritol, and sucralose into melted butter; pour over nut mixture and stir to coat. Spread granola in a single layer on a baking sheet.
- Bake in the preheated oven until crunchy, 8 to 10 minutes. Remove from oven; stir and allow to cool.

Nutrition Info

Per Serving: 183 calories   18.3 g fat

4.3 g carbohydrates   3 g protein

8 mg cholesterol   23 mg sodium

90 Chewy Keto Chocolate Cookies

Prep/Cook Time: 23 m

15 servings

Ingredients

- 1 1/2 cups almond butter
- 2 eggs
- 1/2 cup low-calorie natural sweetener (such as Swerve)
- 1/3 cup unsweetened cocoa powder, sifted
- 1 teaspoon sugar-free vanilla extract
- 1 pinch salt

Instructions

- Preheat oven to 350 degrees F (175 degrees C). Line a baking sheet with parchment paper.

- Combine almond butter, eggs, sweetener, cocoa powder, vanilla extract, and salt in the bowl of a food processor; pulse until a dough forms.
- Roll dough into 1-inch balls. Place on the prepared baking sheet and press down twice with a fork in a criss-cross pattern.
- Bake in the preheated oven until edges are firm, about 12 minutes. Cool on the baking sheet for 1 minute before removing to a wire rack to cool completely.

Nutrition Info

Per Serving: 173 calories	15.7 g fat
12.9 g carbohydrates	5 g protein
25 mg cholesterol	133 mg sodium

91 Loaded Chicken Salad

A delicious salad filled with plenty of vegetables and delicious grilled meat!

Prep Time 10 minutes
Cook Time 8 minutes
Total Time 18 minutes
Servings 4 people

Ingredients

- 1 boneless chicken breast (about 300g, with or without skin)
- 1 tbsp extra virgin olive oil
- 1/4 tsp Himalayan salt

- 1/4 tsp black pepper
- 1 avocado
- 100 g mozzarella balls
- 1 large tomato (any colour)
- 1 har artichoke hearts (my jar was 170g)
- 1/2 red onion
- 5 asparagus
- 20 leaves basil
- 4 cups baby spinach (I used about 200g)

Dressing

- 2 tbsp extra virgin olive oil
- 1 1/2 tbsp balsamic vinegar
- 1 tsp dijon mustard
- 1 clove garlic
- pinch Himalayan salt
- pinch black pepper

Instructions

- Peel and dice the avocado. Slice the red onion. Dice the tomato. Pile the basil leaves together, roll them up and slice. Cut the stems off the asparagus and slice in half. Mince the garlic.
- Slice the chicken breast in half lengthwise. Sprinkle the 1/4 tsp of salt and pepper on each sides. Heat the 1 tbsp of olive oil in a cast iron skillet and place the chicken breasts in. Fry on each side, about 3 minutes each side, until they have a nice golden brown colour and cooked through. Add the asparagus beside the chicken breasts and cook a few minutes until soft and grilled. Take out the chicken and slice.

- In a small bowl, combine the minced garlic, olive oil, balsamic vinegar, dijon, and salt & peper.
- Add the baby spinach to a large bowl or plate. Cover with the grilled chicken, avocado, mozzarella, tomatoes, artichoke, red onions, asparagus and basil leaves. Pour the dressing over and enjoy!

Nutrition Info

Calories 430	Calories from Fat 264
Total Fat 29.36g 45%	Saturated Fat 6.57g 33%
Cholesterol 76mg 25%	Sodium 555mg 23%
Total Carbohydrates 12.86g 4%	Dietary Fiber 6.12g 24%
Sugars 3.16g	Protein 31.73g 63%

92 Easy Shrimp Avocado Salad with Tomatoes and Feta

A delicious and healthy cold shrimp salad with avocado, tomatoes, feta cheese, and lemon juice.

Prep Time 15 minutes
Cook Time 5 minutes
Servings 2 servings

Ingredients

- 8 ounces shrimp peeled, deveined, patted dry
- 1 large avocado diced
- 1 small beefsteak tomato diced and drained
- 1/3 cup crumbled feta cheese

- 1/3 cup freshly chopped cilantro or parsley
- 2 tablespoons salted butter melted
- 1 tablespoon lemon juice
- 1 tablespoon olive oil
- 1/4 teaspoon salt
- 1/4 teaspoon black pepper

Instructions

- Toss shrimp with melted butter in a bowl until well-coated.
- Heat a pan over medium-high heat for a few minutes until hot. Add shrimp to the pan in a single layer, searing for a minute or until it starts to become pink around the edges, then flip and cook until shrimp are cooked through, less than a minute.
- Transfer the shrimp to a plate as they finish cooking. Let them cool while you prepare the other ingredients.
- Add all other ingredients to a large mixing bowl -- diced avocado, diced tomato, feta cheese, cilantro, lemon juice, olive oil, salt, and pepper -- and toss to mix.
- Add shrimp and stir to mix together. Add additional salt and pepper to taste.

Nutrition Info

Calories 430

Total Fat 33g 50%

Sodium 1250mg 52%

Potassium 600mg 17%

Total Carb 12.5g 4%

Protein 24g

93 Keto Chicken Enchilada Bowl

This Keto Chicken Enchilada Bowl is a low carb twist on a Mexican favorite! It's SO easy to make, totally filling and ridiculously yummy!

Prep Time: 20 minutes
Cook Time: 30 minutes
Total Time: 50 minutes
4 servings

Ingredients

- 2 tablespoons coconut oil (for searing chicken)
- 1 pound of boneless, skinless chicken thighs
- 3/4 cup red enchilada sauce (recipe from Low Carb Maven)
- 1/4 cup water
- 1/4 cup chopped onion
- 1– 4 oz can diced green chiles

Toppings (feel free to customize)

- 1 whole avocado, diced
- 1 cup shredded cheese (I used mild cheddar)
- 1/4 cup chopped pickled jalapenos
- 1/2 cup sour cream
- 1 roma tomato, chopped

Optional: serve over plain cauliflower rice (or mexican cauliflower rice) for a more complete meal!

Instructions

- In a pot or dutch oven over medium heat melt the coconut oil. Once hot, sear chicken thighs until lightly brown.
- Pour in enchilada sauce and water then add onion and green chiles. Reduce heat to a simmer and cover. Cook chicken for 17-25 minutes or until chicken is tender and fully cooked through to at least 165 degrees internal temperature.
- Careully remove the chicken and place onto a work surface. Chop or shred chicken (your preference) then add it back into the pot. Let the chicken simmer uncovered for an additional 10 minutes to absorb flavor and allow the sauce to reduce a little.
- To Serve, top with avocado, cheese, jalapeno, sour cream, tomato, and any other desired toppings. Feel free to customize these to your preference. Serve alone or over cauliflower rice if desired just be sure to update your personal nutrition info as needed.

Nutrition Info

Serving Size: 1/4 recipe yield
Calories: 568 Calories
Fat: 40.21g
Carbohydrates: 6.14g NET Carbs
Protein: 38.38g

94 Roasted Lemon Butter Garlic Shrimp and Asparagus

Prep Time: 10 minutes
Cook Time: 12 minutes
Servings:6

Ingredients

Asparagus

- 1 pound thin/medium asparagus ends trimmed
- 1 tablespoon olive oil
- 1 garlic clove, minced
- 1/4 teaspoon salt
- 1/8 teaspoon pepper

Shrimp

- 1 1/2 pounds medium uncooked peeled shrimp deveined*
- 1 tablespoon olive oil
- 2-3 garlic cloves, minced
- 1/2 teaspoon salt
- 1/4 teaspoon paprika
- 1/8 teaspoon pepper
- 1/8-1/4 teaspoon red pepper flakes
- 3 tablespoons chopped fresh parsley
- 1 1/2 tablespoons lemon juice or more to taste
- 3 tablespoons butter, cubed

Serve with

- Pasta
- Rice

Instructions

- Preheat oven to 400 degrees F.
- Line a Jelly Roll Pan (10x15) with foil and lightly spray with cooking spray. Add asparagus and drizzle with 1 tablespoon olive oil. Add 1 minced garlic clove, 1/4 teaspoon salt and 1/8 teaspoon pepper. Toss until evenly coated then line asparagus in a single layer. Roast for 4-6 minutes depending on thickness.
- Meanwhile, remove tails from shrimp.
- Remove pan from oven and push asparagus to one side of the pan (keep in a single layer). Add shrimp and drizzle with 1 tablespoon olive oil. Add 2-3 minced garlic cloves (or more to taste), 1/2 teaspoon salt, 1/4 teaspoon paprika, 1/8 teaspoon pepper, 1/8-1/4 teaspoon red chili flakes and fresh parsley. Toss until evenly coated then line shrimp in a single layer.
- Top asparagus with 1 tablespoon cubed butter, evenly spaced. Top shrimp with 2 tablespoons cubed butter, evenly spaced. Roast for 6 minutes or just until shrimp is opaque.
- Remove pan from oven and drizzle with lemon juice. Season with additional salt and pepper to taste. Serve with pasta, rice, etc.

95 Caprese Eggplant Panini with Lemon Basil Aioli

Serves: 2-4

Ingredients

- 2 Small Eggplants, ends removed
- 2 cloves Garlic, peeled
- 2 tbsp Mayonnaise
- 8-10 Lemon Basil leaves, chopped
- ½ cup Mozzarella, shredded
- 2 small Tomatoes, campari or other petite variety
- 1 cup Spinach Leaves
- 2 tbsp Toasted Pine Nuts

Instructions

- Heat a panini press (or countertop grill with closable lid) to medium.
- Remove ends of each small (baby) eggplant and slice in half, cutting end to end. Slice the remaining eggplant in ½ inch pieces and discard any pieces that are mostly skin.
- In a hot skillet, brown garlic cloves until fragrant and soft. Once cool, mince garlic and add to mayonnaise. Stir in chopped lemon basil to finish the aioli.

Assemble panini

- Spread aioli onto an eggplant slice and top with spinach leaves, tomato slices, fresh mozzarella and pine nuts. Spread more aioli on another eggplant slice and place ontop. Grill until cheese is melted. Serve hot!

96 Cinnamon Pork Chops & Mock Apples

Hearty, healthy, and delicious, cinnamon pork chops with chayote mock apples makes a fantastic family dinner or meal prep for the work week!

Prep Time 5 minutes   Cook Time 40 minutes
Total Time 45 minutes   Servings 4

Ingredients

- 2 tbsp ghee
- 1/2 tsp sea salt
- 4 pork chops boneless
- 2 chayote chopped to 1/2-inch chunks
- 2 tbsp monkfruit sweetener or low carb sweetener of choice
- 1 tsp cinnamon
- 1/8 tsp nutmeg
- 1 tbsp apple cider vinegar

Instructions

- Melt ghee in a large skillet over medium heat, add pork chops and cook for 5 minutes.
- Flip the pork chops and add chayote and sprinkle sweetener, cinnamon, nutmeg, and apple cider vinegar over the top. Cook for an additional 4-5 minutes, or until the pork chops reach the appropriate temperature (145 F for medium rare, 160 for medium).

- Remove the pork chops and place in a meal prep container if preparing meals for the week, otherwise keep pork chops warm until ready to serve.
- Bring the chayote mixture to a boil for several minutes. Reduce heat to low medium and simmer with cover, stirring occasionally, for 30 to 40 minutes. When done, the chayote will be fork tender and similar in texture to baked apple.
- Divide the chayote mock apples between four meal prep containers or serve immediately alongside the warm pork chops.

Nutrition Info

Calories 288

Calories from Fat 144

Total Fat 16g 25%

Saturated Fat 7g 35%

Cholesterol 108mg 36%

Sodium 356mg 15%

Potassium 582mg 17%

Total Carbohydrates 3g 1%

Dietary Fiber 1g 4%

Sugars 1g

Protein 29g 58%

97 Spicy Kimchi Ahi Poke

Prep 10 mins

Total 10 mins

Yield 4 portions

Ingredients

- 1 lb sushi-grade ahi tuna, diced to roughly 1 inch
- 1 tbsp soy sauce (or Coconut Aminos for Paleo)

- 1/2 tsp sesame oil
- 1/4 cup mayo
- 2 tbsp sriracha (PaleoChef makes a Paleo-friendly version)
- 1 ripe avocado, diced
- 1/2 cup kimchi
- chopped green onion
- sesame seeds

Instructions

- In a medium mixing bowl, add diced tuna.
- Add soy sauce, sesame oil, mayo, sriracha to the bowl and toss to combine.
- Add diced avocado and kimchi to the bowl and gently combine.
- Serve on top of salad greens, cauli rice, or traditional rice and top with a sprinkle of chopped green onion and sesame seeds if desired.

Nutrition Info

Serving Size 1 portion	Calories 299
Total Fat 18 g	Saturated Fat 2 g
Cholesterol 70 mg	Sodium 431 mg
Total Carbohydrates 5 g	Protein 5 g

98 Low Carb Chicken Philly Cheesesteak

Family friendly low carb chicken philly cheesesteak comes together in a snap. Serve in bowls for the low carb eaters and on a hoagie bun for everyone else.

Prep Time: 10 minutes
Cook Time: 15 minutes
Total Time: 25 minutes
Servings: 3

Ingredients

- 10 oz boneless chicken breasts (about 2)
- 2 Tbsp worcestershire sauce
- 1/2 tsp onion powder
- 1/2 tsp garlic powder
- 1 dash ground pepper
- 2 tsp olive oil, divided
- 1/2 cup diced onion fresh or frozen
- 1/2 cup diced bell pepper fresh or frozen
- 1/2 tsp minced garlic
- 3 slices provolone cheese or queso melting cheese

Instructions

- Slice chicken breasts into very thin pieces (freeze slightly if desired to make this easier) and place in a medium bowl. Add next 4 ingredients (worcestershire through ground pepper) and stir to coat chicken.

- Heat 1 teaspoon olive oil in a large (9") oven proof skillet. Add chicken pieces and cook until browned -about 5 minutes. Turn pieces over and cook about 2-3 minutes more or until brown. Remove from skillet.
- Add remaining 1 teaspoon olive oil to warm skillet. Then add onions, bell pepper and garlic. Cook and stir to heated and tender- 2-3 minutes.
- Turn heat off and add chicken back to skillet and stir with veggies to combine. Place sliced cheese over all and cover 2-3 minutes to melt.

Note:

Serve up in bowls for those eating low carb. Serve with warm hoagie rolls for others.

Nutrition Info

Calories: 263kcal

Protein: 27g

Saturated Fat: 5g

Sodium: 330mg

Fiber: 1g, Sugar: 2g

Carbohydrates: 5g

Fat: 13g

Cholesterol: 79mg

Potassium: 570mg

99 Easy Asiago Cauliflower Rice (low carb)

Prep Time 15 minutes
Cook Time 10 minutes
Total Time 25 minutes
Servings 4

Ingredients

- 3 cups cauliflower riced
- 1 cup Asiago cheese shredded
- 3/4 cup heavy cream

Instructions

- In a large saute pan, add the riced cauliflower and 2 tablespoons of water. Cover and cook for 5 minutes.
- Add the cream and cheese and mix until cheese is melted.
- Taste to see if the cauliflower is done.
- Take off the heat and serve.

100 Spinach-Mozzarella Stuffed Burgers

4 people

Ingredients

- 1½ lbs ground chuck
- 1 teaspoon salt
- ¾ teaspoon ground black pepper
- 2 cups fresh spinach, firmly packed

- ½ cup shredded mozzarella cheese (about 4 oz)
- 2 tablespoons grated Parmesan cheese

Instructions

- In a medium bowl, combine ground beef, salt, and pepper.
- Scoop about ?cup of mixture and with dampened hands shape into 8 patties about ½-inch thick. Place in the refrigerator.
- Place spinach in saucepan over medium-high heat. Cover and cook for 2 minutes, until wilted.
- Drain and let cool. With your hands squeeze the spinach to extract as much liquid as possible.
- Transfer to a cutting board, chop the spinach, and place in a bowl.
- Stir in mozzarella cheese and Parmesan.
- Scoop about ¼ cup of stuffing and mound in the center of 4 patties,
- Cover with remaining 4 patties, and seal the edges by pressing firmly together.
- Cup each patty with your hands to round out the edges, and press on the top to flatten slightly into a single thick patty.
- Heat a grill or a grill pan to medium-high (if you're using an outdoor grill lightly oil the grill grates).
- Grill burgers for 5 to 6 minutes on each side.
- Serve!

Nutrition Info

One patty yields 414 calories   29 grams of fat
1 gram of carbs   36 grams of protein.

CONCLUSION

Selecting the right food will be easier as you become accustomed to the Keto approach. Instead of lean meats, you'll focus on skin-on poultry, fattier parts like chicken thighs, rib-eye steaks, grass-fed ground beef, fattier fish like salmon, beef brisket or pork shoulder, and bacon. Leafy greens such as spinach, kale and lettuce, along with broccoli, cauliflower and cucumbers, make healthy vegetable choices (but you'll avoid starchy root foods like carrots, potatoes, turnips and parsnips). You can work in less-familiar veggies such as kohlrabi or daikon.

Oils like avocado, olive, canola, flaxseed and palm, as well as mayonnaise will flavor salads while fattening them up. Clarified butter, or ghee, is a fat you'll use for cooking or as a spread.

Our responses to the ketogenic diet are individualized. They're based on our biology, our metabolism, our numbers and the way we feel.

Some people can sustain the diet for decades. Others don't do well on it.

If you happen to be very thin, if you have an eating disorder, or if you have certain metabolic issues, the keto diet will also be risky for you. Be very careful; check with your doctor before trying this diet.

www.ingramcontent.com/pod-product-compliance
Lightning Source LLC
Chambersburg PA
CBHW060507290526
45791CB00001B/303